DISEASES
IN HISTORY

Plague

Diseases in History

PLAGUE

Kevin Cunningham

MORGAN REYNOLDS

PUBLISHING

Greensboro, North Carolina

Diseases in History

PLAGUE

FLU

MALARIA

HIV/AIDS

Library of Congress Cataloging-in-Publication Data

Cunningham, Kevin, 1966-
Diseases in history. Plague / by Kevin Cunningham.
p. cm.
Includes bibliographical references and index.
ISBN-13: 978-1-59935-102-5
ISBN-10: 1-59935-102-1
1. Plague--History. I. Title. II. Title: Plague.
RC172.C86 2009
614.5'732--dc22
                    2008051618

Printed in the United States of America
First Edition

Contents

Introduction

*I*t was said the plague came from the East.

Manchurians feared its onset in the autumn, recognized it came from the furry rodents they hunted for food and fur, and learned to avoid the sick animals staggering about in a silence unusual for such social creatures. Fierce steppe peoples like the Mongols, conquerors of countless human foes, fell to it. The Islamic world accepted it as the will of Allah. Christian Europe blamed it on the anger of God.

Medieval Europeans did not call it the Black Death. To them it was the *pest*, as in pestilence. When it returned in 1347, it unleashed a holocaust that in four years killed a third—or possibly half, possibly two-thirds—of Europe's population. It probably did the same to the Muslim countries and to those on the caravan routes across the Central Asian steppe. China may have suffered even greater loss of life.

Nothing stopped plague. Very little provided comfort. Giovanni Boccaccio, a witness to the Black Death in Florence, wrote, "It was proof against all human providence and remedies, such as the appointment of officials to the task of ridding the city of much refuse, the banning of sick visitors from outside, and a good number of sanitary ordinances; equally unavailing were the humble petitions offered to the Lord by pious souls not once but countless times. . . ."

The word "plague" likely comes from the Greek *plaga*, meaning a blow or a strike, as in being hit by a strong force. To the Greeks, and to other ancient peoples borrowing their word, *plaga* referred to epidemics in general, just as the word plague does for many people today. It was centuries later that "plague" also came to mean a specific disease caused by the rod-shaped bacterium *Yersinia pestis*. When this book refers to plague, it means that specific disease.

Plague was (and is), for the most part, a rodent disease. But at three times in recorded history it has crossed over to the human population and caused a pandemic—a series of epidemics that strikes large areas of the world. In the case of plague, the epidemics returned in wave after wave for centuries. The Third Pandemic continues today in countries as diverse as India, the Democratic Republic of Congo, and the United States.

Few if any diseases have inspired so much dread, or so much art. From the medieval era onward, painters created countless images of Grim Reapers and skeletal pest maidens spreading the disease across the sky. Daniel Defoe, the author of *Robinson Crusoe*, penned *A Journal of the Plague-Year* about the Great Plague of London (1665), an event he survived. More than two hundred years later, Albert Camus's novel *The Plague* used an epidemic in Algeria as a launching point to study the human condition. The disease even foiled Juliet's plans to reunite with Romeo.

So fearsome was its power to kill that the phrase "bubonic plague" causes panic to this day. And that's despite the fact that the disease is treatable with antibiotics and that today only some one thousand to 3,000 cases appear worldwide each year.

Plague lingers in many parts of the world and threatens to extend its reach further. Evolutionary processes have shaped it to infect a family of animals that have adapted to virtually any climate and a wide range of habitats. It is one of the few families of animals, in fact, that thrives in proximity to man: the rodents.

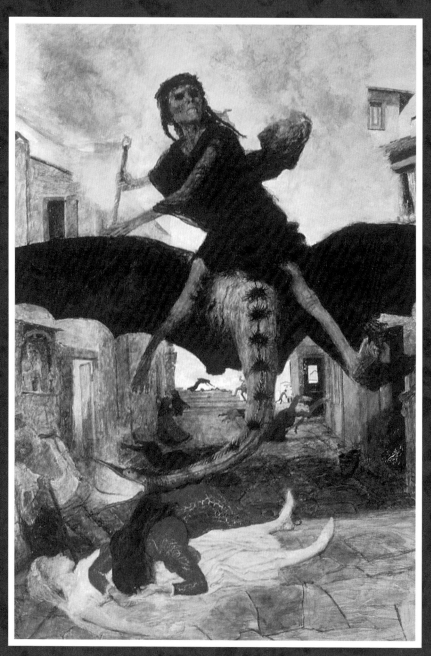

This 1898 painting by Arnold Böcklin personifies the plague as a figure on a dragon, killing its victims in the street.

one
Rats, Fleas, and Plague

Although scientists do not yet understand all the dynamics, it appears that *Yersinia pestis*, the plague bacteria, is always with us—or, at least, always within certain populations of wild rodents in various parts of the world. Within these wild rodent populations, the bacteria continually cycle between the rodents and the fleas that feed on them without causing widespread mortality. Some varieties of wild rodents, it seems, have at least some resistance to the bacteria's deadly effects and, instead of succumbing to plague, serve as reservoirs of plague bacteria between human outbreaks. Every once in a while, however, plague bacteria escape this cozy cycle and infect rodent populations that have little or no natural immunity to them. It's unclear exactly why this happens. Environmental changes and even natural disasters may affect the wild rodents' typical food supply or habitat, sending them in search of "greener pastures." And that

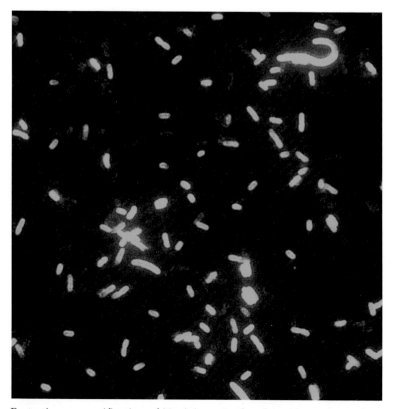

Forty times magnification of *Yersinia pestis*, the plague bacteria
(Courtesy of Larry Stauffer, Oregon State Public Health Laboratory)

search may bring them into contact with rodents that aren't immune to plague, thus providing their fleas with new hosts, and the plague with new victims. If the plague bacteria happen to land on rodents that naturally live in close proximity to humans—namely, rats—many of those new plague victims are likely to be human.

Rats—perhaps the most recognized member of the rodent family—have not only adapted to life among human beings, they prosper by it. Chernobyl offers a vivid example. In 1986, a catastrophic accident at the nuclear plant at Chernobyl,

Ukraine, forced the government to evacuate the area. It remained off-limits two decades later. The region's wildlife has increased in the absence of human beings, despite the presence of radioactive contamination. Wolves, deer, and many kinds of migrating birds have returned to the area.

But not the rats. They need people to provide garbage and sewage.

For centuries, when Europeans complained about rats, they meant the black rat, known by the scientific name *Rattus rattus*. The body of an adult black rat averages six to eight-and-a-half inches long and its tail adds at least that many inches to the animal's total length. Though called the black rat, its fur can also be gray or tan. In the wild, it builds its nests in trees and bushes. Like many rodents, it is social, sleeping in a pile with others and often crawling under a stranger in greeting.

The species evolved as a tree climber in southern Asia. Black rats can climb a ninety-degree vertical surface and have been known to survive five-story falls. In the past, they often nested in the attics and ceilings of houses. *Rattus rattus* also enjoyed life scampering about the complex rigging on sailing ships.

It's unclear when the black rat made its way to Europe. Perhaps it came on ships trading with India, or to Africa by the same method and from there to Europe. It's possible the black rat lived (and died) at Pompeii, putting it in Italy before the city's destruction in AD 79. Or it could have arrived later. All we know for certain is that it eventually spread across the continent.

Many other species of rodent carry plague, as well. One is the black rat's cousin, the brown or Norway rat (*Rattus norvegicus*), a misnamed species originally from northern China.

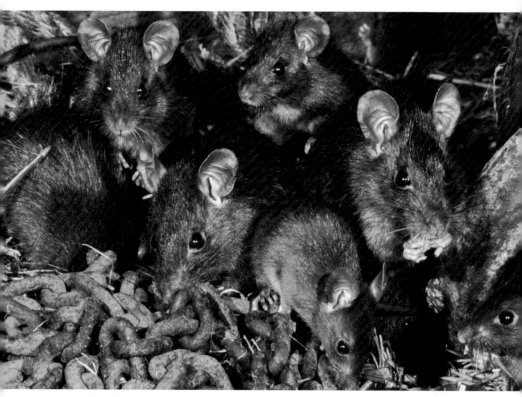

The black rat is one of many rodent species that can carry and spread the plague bacteria. *(Courtesy of Terry Whittaker/Alamy)*

During the 1700s, the brown rat replaced the black in the temperate and cold regions of Europe and North America.

In central Asia, plague spreads via many rodent species, notably several kinds of marmot, an animal valued for its pelt. The plague circulates through several Indian species, including the hefty greater bandicoot rat.

Gerbils carry it in Africa and the Middle East, and Africans must also deal with the plague-carrying multimammate rat, a house pest that breeds at extraordinary rates.

In South America, the disease infects guinea pigs. Plague infects many rodents in North America and is thought to be a major factor in the dwindling of the prairie dog population in the western United States.

Plague, in fact, strikes rodents far more than it strikes humans. They get it from infected fleas. At least thirty and perhaps more than one hundred of the thousands of flea species are capable of carrying the disease, including the human flea, *Pulex irritans*. But natural selection has forged a special relationship between the *Y. pestis* bacterium and one kind of flea in particular.

The Oriental rat flea, or *Xenopsylla cheopis*, acts as the primary vector in the plague cycle. A vector is an insect or other organism that carries a disease-causing agent and transmits it to humans or another animal species.

As its name implies, the Oriental rat flea prefers to live on rodents. It takes in plague bacteria while feeding on the blood of an infected rodent host. Often the flea lives on unaffected. But occasionally the bacteria breeds inside it and blocks the flea's digestive system. As the flea begins to starve, it goes into a feeding frenzy, biting wherever it can as often as it can.

Xenopsylla cheopis, the Oriental rat flea, extracting blood from its host. The Oriental rat flea acts as the primary vector in the plague cycle. (*Courtesy of World Health Organization*)

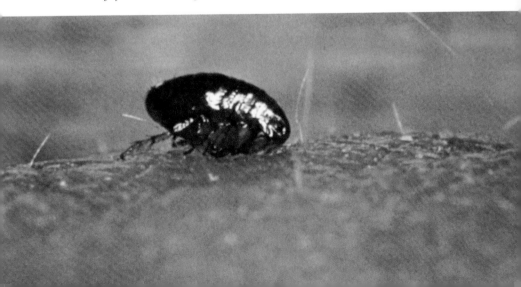

With each bite, it regurgitates thousands of plague bacteria into the animal it is trying to feed upon.

If plague kills the rodent host before the flea starves to death, *X. cheopis* hops off the dead rat and attaches itself to the nearest host. Usually it's easy to find another—in many rodent species, the animals flock together in colonies. But living hosts can be hard to come by during times of plague. If unable to find a rodent, the flea looks for a substitute. Many warm-blooded mammals will do—including human beings.

Many kinds of bacteria that enter the human body through wounds tend to first cluster around the entry site, where special cells employed by the body's immune system can more easily track them down, contain them, and destroy them. But the safety-pin-shaped *Y. pestis* has evolved to hide from mammalian immune systems. Special enzymes prevent clustering, allowing the bacteria to evade the body's first line of defense. *Y. pestis* is also skilled at tricking the immune system into thinking it is harmless. It even prevents the initial inflammation that serves as one of the body's most important internal warning signals of infection. A short time later, the mammal develops plague.

Few diseases match the lethality of untreated plague. It is at least as deadly as smallpox. Even severe strains of influenza do not approach the bubonic form's death rate. And bubonic plague is the mild form.

"So far we have not found any single thing that makes this bacteria so virulent," said the Russian plague expert Vladimir Motin. "[I]t's the combination of many different factors, all of which are also present in other pathogens. Somehow evolution selected for the right combinations to make this thing dedicated to kill."

Adding to plague's mystique is the fact that this one disease can appear in three major forms: bubonic, septicemic, and pneumonic. Each form presents different symptoms, attacks different parts of the body, and spreads in different ways.

Bubonic plague occurs when a flea infected with *Y. pestis* bites a human being. Less often the bacteria enters the body through a break in the skin or, in rare cases, when a victim eats an infected animal.

Y. pestis bacteria then head for the nearest lymph nodes— in the neck, armpits, or groin—and from there move to the liver and spleen. Once established, the bacteria breed in explosive numbers.

Bubonic plague symptoms usually appear two to six days after the flea bite. Fever and chills wrack the body. Headache is common. There's also extreme and unexplained exhaustion. Because these symptoms accompany many other illnesses as well, plague can be hard to diagnose.

Within a day or so after the first symptoms appear, hemorrhaging causes the lymph nodes to bulge into the telltale *bubo*. The bubo typically measures one to ten centimeters across. Often it is hot to the touch. Swollen purple splotches ring the bubo as blood collects under the skin. Moving the area at all causes excruciating pain. Sometimes tissue and muscle around the bubo blackens and rots away. On occasion a bubo will burst, releasing foul-smelling pus.

An advanced case can bring on delirium, shock, and coma. Old texts mention high fever and hallucinations. Left untreated, bubonic plague kills between 50 and 60 percent of the time. Survivors often experience plague-related fatigue for weeks or months afterward.

Pneumonic plague is a rare form of the disease. It affects the lungs, causing a kind of extreme pneumonia. Primary pneumonic plague spreads through the air, when bacteria-carrying droplets are coughed or sneezed out by an infected person and breathed in by others, infecting them in turn. Secondary pneumonic plague starts out as bubonic plague that spreads to the lungs.

A person inhaling infected droplets experiences symptoms within one to six days; most often they appear two to four days after contact, although they can start within hours. There is a sudden onset of high fever, weakness, and headache punctuated by chest pain, difficulty breathing, and a cough that brings up bloody and/or frothy sputum. In some cases, the victim also experiences abdominal pain, nausea, vomiting, and diarrhea.

Massive amounts of fluid fill the lungs. Hemorrhaging takes place. Cardiovascular collapse strikes with overwhelming force. Unless treated, pneumonic plague kills close to 100 percent of its victims, ranking it among the deadliest of contagious human diseases. Death occurs quickly once symptoms appear—often two to four but sometimes up to six days after the initial contact.

An uncommon condition called septicemic plague occurs when the plague bacteria infect the blood instead of or after attacking the lymphatic system. It can develop as a complication of bubonic plague or, like bubonic plague, it can occur through the bite of a plague-infected flea. Bacteria levels in the bloodstream can quickly skyrocket to such high levels that even non-plague-carrying insects like lice can take in *Y. pestis* by biting the victim.

Without fast antibiotic treatment, septicemic plague is always fatal. Some victims of septicemic plague die before symptoms even have a chance to appear. When symptoms do appear, the victim typically has no more than about fifteen hours to live. Symptoms include fever and chills; weakness; abdominal pain; bleeding from the nose, mouth, and/or rectum; internal bleeding from organs and bleeding under the skin; shock; and gangrene (blackening and death) in the extremities. Even those who get treatment in time are vulnerable to severe gangrene in the tissues of the nose, fingers, and toes.

Yersinia pestis is thought to have evolved at least 1,500 and possibly as long as 20,000 years ago from another, less harmful bacterium found in the intestinal system. Scientists can only speculate where it originated. The majority opinion places the origin in the steppe region of central Asia—perhaps Manchuria, perhaps Mongolia, perhaps nearby but further west.

As ancient civilizations formed, conditions developed that encouraged the plague bacterium to spread to new lands. Human beings from one part of the world increasingly came into contact with those from far away. The diverse peoples exchanged many things. Exotic goods. Blows with swords. And diseases.

Notable Plague Epidemics in History

Location	Date(s)	Estimated number of deaths
Constantinople, "Plague of Justinian"	AD 542	60,000
Europe, Egypt, Persia	AD 541-547	Unknown; millions
Europe, "Black Death"	1347-1351	25 million
China	1330s-1400	Unknown; millions
Europe, *Pestis Secundus*	Early 1360s	Unknown; millions
London, "Great Plague"	1665-1666	100,000
Russian Empire	1770-1772	127,000+
Canton, China	1880s	70,000
Hong Kong	1894	2500+
India	1896-1910	10 million
San Francisco	1907	77
Manchuria	1910-1911	60,000
Changten, China	1941	7,643
Surat, India	1994	54

two

Justinian's Plague

Diseases evolved in specific areas, just as plant and animal species did. Over time, the disease-causing pathogen (such as a virus, bacterium, or parasite) became a part of an area's ecosystem and adapted to the species that carried it and caught it. In some cases, the pathogen evolved into a less lethal form before it wiped out the host species it needed.

An area where a specific pathogen evolved and developed relationships with local organisms (including humans) was what the historian William McNeill referred to as a disease pool. The steppe region (and disease pool) of Manchuria had its own pathogens. So did the lands ringing the Mediterranean Sea. And so on.

Human societies in a particular disease pool continually encountered pathogens that were endemic—present in their area on a permanent basis. In the early period of human history, an endemic disease remained within the disease pool where it evolved. Several possible factors kept it from spreading. Natural features, like the Himalayas or an ocean, contained it. If the animal that transmitted the pathogen could not survive the climate of an adjacent ecosystem, the disease could not trespass into it. The limits of human travel also restricted it, since travel is a way humans often spread their diseases.

Disease pools began to overlap as ancient peoples came into contact with each other. China, Central Asia, and India had mutual contact via missionaries and trade. Ships linked Egypt's Nile region with Greece, while Greek armies and merchants ventured into the Middle East, Persia, and Armenia. Greece's expansion into an empire brought parts of western Europe and Africa's Mediterranean coast into the picture.

For the first time in history, there were semipermanent contacts between peoples from different disease pools. The people from each carried their endemic pathogens faster and farther than before, thanks to road systems and more reliable shipping routes.

Records remain too incomplete to help us make an accurate list of ancient epidemics. We know the so-called Plague of Athens—possibly the bacterial disease typhus—struck Greece in 430 BC. But, from the evidence we have at this time, it appears large-scale outbreaks of diseases brought to Mediterranean Europe from distant disease pools first became a true danger during the time of the Roman Empire.

In AD 251, the so-called Antonine Plague broke out in the empire. It appears to have been either measles or smallpox, brought back from Mesopotamia by Roman soldiers. The

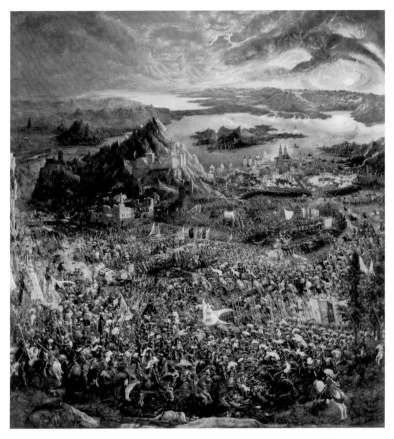

Greece's military expansion led to people from different disease pools coming into contact with each other for the first time in history. In this 1529 painting, the ancient Greek army, commanded by Alexander the Great, battles Persian forces in Anatolia. *(Courtesy of Getty Images)*

Romans, lacking immunity to the pathogen, died in huge numbers. Writers of the time placed the peak death toll at 5,000 a day in the city of Rome. Some historians believe that the population losses, combined with disruptions in trade, may have contributed to the empire's slow decline.

Measles arrived either as the Antonine Plague or as another invading pathogen during the same period. As it became a

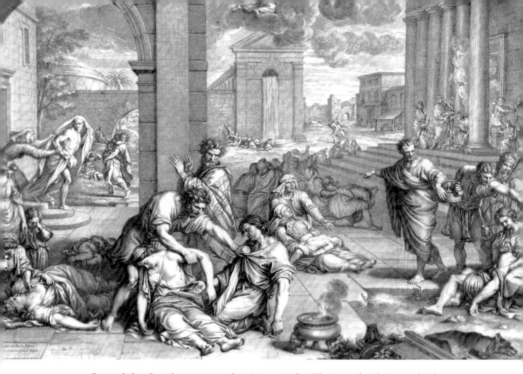

One of the first known epidemics was the Plague of Athens, which struck Greece in 430 BC. *(Library of Congress)*

part of the Mediterranean disease pool, however, measles underwent a transformation. Like many diseases, it confers lifelong immunity to anyone who survives it. So new outbreaks in the Mediterranean harmed only those lacking immunity, i.e., those never exposed before, most of whom were children born since the last epidemic. Measles, a killer of adults during the Roman Empire, gradually turned into a common (if deadly) childhood illness. Smallpox underwent a similar change.

Exactly when and how *Y. pestis* first escaped its original disease pool is unknown. It may have arrived in Mongolia and Manchuria in prehistory, assuming it did not evolve there. In ancient times it traveled over the Himalayas to India, where it found amenable rodent hosts like the black rat. From India it may have leapt to Africa via ships, though at what point that occurred (if it did) remains uncertain.

We do know, however, that bubonic plague struck Mediterranean Europe in the sixth century. The resulting disaster surpassed even those brought by smallpox and measles. Historians called it Justinian's Plague, after the Byzantine emperor of the time.

The western Roman Empire, based in Rome, had fallen apart during the 400s. Armies of Goths, Ostrogoths, Huns, and other peoples had warred up and down the Italian peninsula ever since. Across the Adriatic Sea, however, the Byzantine, or Eastern, Empire flourished. Constantinople, its capital, was among the largest and richest cities in the world.

In 527, the empire came under the leadership of Justinian. The new emperor possessed a far-ranging mind and tremendous energy. His overriding ambition was to recapture Italy and rebuild the Roman Empire of old. He began a long series of wars, not just in Italy, but against the competing Persian Empire in the East. Wars cost money, and Justinian taxed heavily. But he had the good fortune of ruling a prosperous trading empire able to provide him with revenue.

Egypt was one of the empire's major trading partners. Constantinople fed its citizens on imported Egyptian grain and imported great amounts of Egyptian cloth. Both may have played a part in bringing bubonic plague to the city—certainly the grain did. The city used four immense warehouses to store it, including one immense building that measured ninety feet across and 280 feet long (its height is unknown). The mountains of grain inside drew swarms of rats and other hungry rodents. The rats, if not other species, harbored *X. cheopis*. To add to the threat, the storehouses offered the flea an excellent breeding ground—*X. cheopis'* young fed on grain and rice dust.

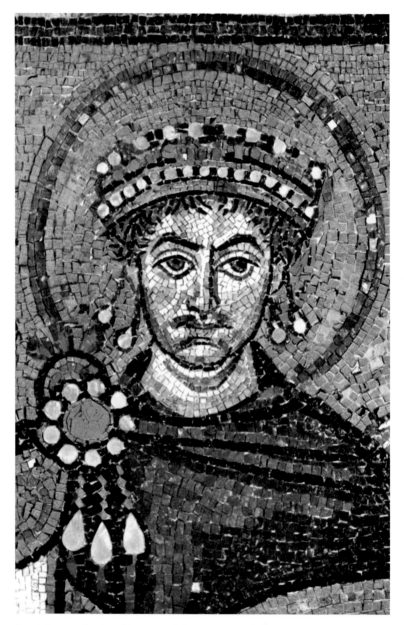

Justinian as depicted in one of the mosaics of the Basilica of San Vitale in Italy

An epidemic of the bubonic form of plague came to Pelusium, in Egypt, in AD 541. It may have arrived there from Ethiopia. Whether it originated in East Africa or arrived on ships from India remains unknown. The disease reached the port of Alexandria shortly after it hit Pelusium and the same year devastated Palestine and Syria.

A 1498 painting of the port of Seville, Spain. The plague has a classic pattern of starting in port cities and then spreading to nearby areas. *(Courtesy of The London Art Archive/Alamy)*

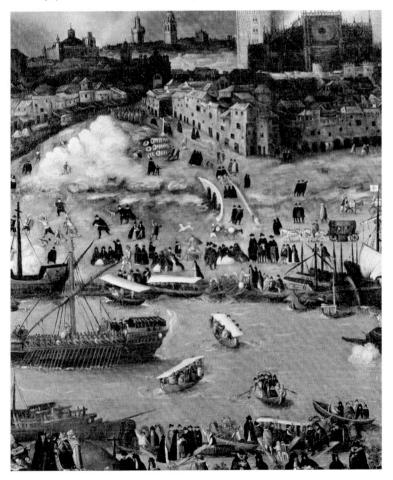

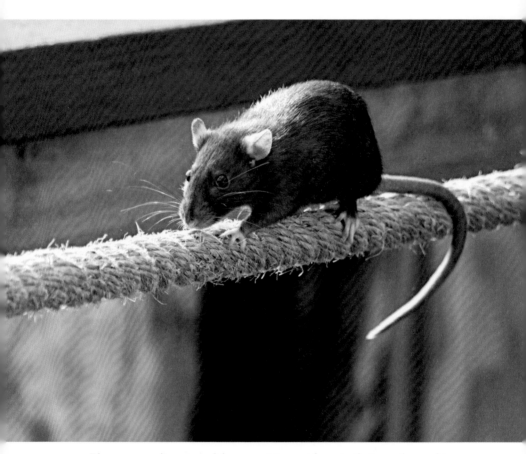

Plague was often spread from port to port by rats that ran down ship ropes into town. *(Courtesy of David Kilpatrick/Alamy)*

The epidemic reached Constantinople late in the year. At first the winter cold kept it under control—*X. cheopis* did not function well in cold weather. But the rats and fleas returned in the spring. From Constantinople bubonic plague sped east into Armenia, Mesopotamia, and Persia and west on board ships bound for Italy.

The plague struck first in port cities and then moved into nearby areas. This came to be recognized as a classic pattern for the spread of bubonic plague. The moment a ship tied off in port, *X. cheopis*-ridden rats ran down the ropes into town. Workers unloading Egyptian cloth were exposed to the disease through the bites of fleas living in the fabric. Thanks to Justinian's troop movements and the empire's commercial prosperity, ships crisscrossed the region in numbers not seen for generations.

One of the epidemic's most terrifying aspects was its unpredictability. Accounts tell of how remote monasteries in one place were wiped out, whereas monasteries in neighboring valleys did not suffer at all. People died of plague in a village in the interior, while another, nearer to the sea, weathered the epidemic unharmed.

The Byzantine historian Procopius witnessed the epidemic in Constantinople and described the bubonic plague symptoms in clinical detail.

> They had a sudden fever, some when just roused from sleep, others while walking about, and others while otherwise engaged, without any regard to what they were doing. And the body showed no change from its previous color, nor was it hot as might be expected when attacked by a fever, nor indeed did any inflammation set in, but the fever was of such a languid sort from its commencement and up till evening that neither to the sick themselves nor to a physician who touched them would it afford any suspicion of danger. . . . But on the same day in some cases, in others on the following day, and in the rest not many days later, a bubonic swelling developed; and this took place not only in the particular part of the body which is called "boubon," [bubo] that is, below the abdomen, but also inside the armpit, and in some cases also beside the ears, and at different points on the thighs.

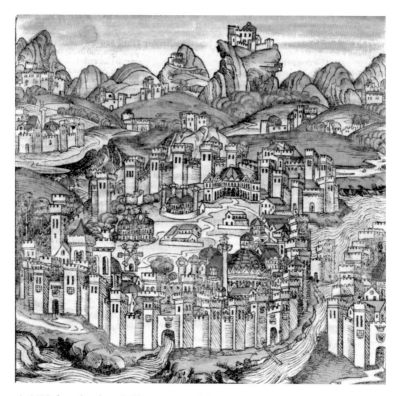

A 1493, hand-colored illustration of Constantinople. During the height of Justinian's Plague, between 5,000 and 10,000 people died every day in Constantinople.

At first Constantinople's death toll was small, the victims hardly noticed. Though the disease initially hit the poor, by late spring of AD 542 it had engulfed all classes, all walks of life. Justinian himself caught it in the summer (and survived).

As the plague gained strength, the authorities took steps to control it. Justinian even ordered his soldiers to put aside their weapons and take control of sanitation.

Even with soldiers collecting the bodies, however, the plague gained strength. The disease was unlike anything the Byzantines had ever seen. How it spread boggled Constantinople's wisest physicians because, clearly, the disease did not pass from person to person. Bacteria, viruses, and parasites remained unknown at that time. That fleas on rats or hiding in cloth caused such a holocaust would have been incomprehensible to them.

The religious explained the disease in their own way. John of Ephesus said, "Thus when the punishment, in which God's abundant kindness and grace were really visible, reached this city, though it was horrible, powerful and intense, we ought to call it not only a threatening sign and wrath but also a sign of mercy and a call for repentance."

Faith helped people fit an inexplicable event like bubonic plague into their worldview. Declaring it to be God's punishment gave it a purpose, at least. It seemed unthinkable that something so horrible could strike without a reason.

Neither medicine, nor prayer, nor the prophecies spun by local seers stopped the plague. Constantinople became a ghost town. Those craftsmen still living fled from their workshops. Businesses closed. Trade came to a halt. Warehouses and markets sat empty.

A grim scene developed in Constantinople, one that would be repeated again and again for more than two centuries and would return on an even wider scale during the Black Death. Throughout the city, soldiers and poor men willing to take the work drove carts piled with corpses. Others lay the dead in mass graves and then pressed down the bodies to make space for the next wave. Bodies on barges were stacked and counted and at last dumped into the sea due to lack of space in the burial pits. But the dead continued to pile up. Bloated corpses burst and oozed up and down the shoreline. City leaders turned to desperate measures:

> . . . but later on those who were making these trenches, no longer able to keep up with the number of the dying, mounted the towers of the fortifications in Sycae, and tearing off the roofs threw the bodies in there in complete disorder; and they piled them up just as each one happened to fall, and filled practically all the towers with corpses, and then covered them again with their roofs. As a result of this an evil stench pervaded the city and distressed the inhabitants still more, and especially whenever the wind blew fresh from that quarter.

Constantinople agonized for four months. According to Procopius, plague killed between 5,000 and 10,000 people every day during the height of the epidemic.

Justinian's Plague burnt itself out in 544. No one knows for sure how many died. Though historians argue about Constantinople's pre-plague population, many put the figure between 250,000 and 300,000. A 20 percent mortality rate would mean that 50,000 to 60,000 people died in the city alone.

The plague did not halt at the city limits of Constantinople. Throughout 543 and 544 the disease spread from Italy to Spain, southern France, and much of Europe south of the Alps. The total death count remains uncertain. Ancient sources have a habit of exaggerating losses in epidemics that rival their exaggerations of deaths on battlefields. The historian J. B. Bury thought it killed a third of the population in some places. Overall, a third of the people of Mediterranean Europe may have died, with an unknown loss of life in Persia, Armenia, and other Eastern countries.

Justinian's Plague showed the power of bubonic plague to alter the course of an empire, even the course of history. The epidemic weakened the Byzantine Empire in every aspect. The government lost a generation of experienced bureaucrats and military leaders and noble families. The economy lost the businessmen and merchants who controlled its trade; sea routes withered for lack of traders and sailors. Once-valuable farmland became fallow, villages were deserted, goats sheltered in abandoned monasteries. Society lost scholars and teachers, physicians and clergymen, skilled artisans and their students.

The deaths of so many taxpayers and the loss of so much profitable trade forced Justinian to cut spending, even military spending. Enemies on all sides moved to take advantage. Though Justinian paid the hated Persians for peace, he soon faced a revolt by his subjects in North Africa. Germanic tribes counterattacked his armies in Italy. Trouble even stirred nearer to home, in the Balkans. The chance to restore the glory of Rome had slipped from the emperor's grasp. Neither Justinian nor his successors would fulfill the dream.

The outbreaks that spread from Pelusium to Constantinople and beyond mark the beginning of what historians call plague's First Pandemic. In the aftermath of Justinian's Plague, *Y. pestis* established itself among the rats and fleas, and bubonic plague became endemic throughout much of Mediterranean Europe, the Middle East, and northern Africa. It returned in cycles. Four more epidemics swept through the region before the end of the sixth century. Seven more hit during the 600s. Outbreaks occasionally took place north of the Alps and even reached as far away as Ireland and Britain.

The First Pandemic sputtered to an end after 767. When plague broke out in Europe after that, it did so as an import brought from other countries. These coastal outbreaks did not spread far. Bubonic plague became lost in history, a half-remembered horror story passed down through generations and recalled here and there by a traveler as she passed the crumbling walls of a monastery, the ruins of an old village, an empty wasteland that was once filled with tall yellow wheat and flowering orchards.

three
The Coming of the Black Death

Europe's climate became drier and warmer for a four hundred year period starting in AD 750 or 800. Both conditions were favorable to agriculture. During the same period, advances in European technology led to increased food production. New plows and harnesses allowed farmers to replace the ox with the horse, a superior work animal. Better windmills and watermills provided a new source of power.

More food curbed health problems related to malnutrition—there were many—and encouraged a higher birthrate. Europe's population, long in decline, rebounded, and continued to do so into the 1100s and 1200s. Though the cities expanded, Europeans remained an overwhelmingly rural people. New villages were founded. Peasants cleared forests for farmland, allowing for still greater food production.

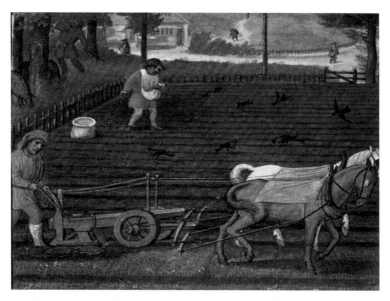

An illustration of a farmer plowing with a team of horses. During the Middle Ages, advances in plowing technology allowed farmers to increase agricultural production.

Then, sometime in the thirteenth century, nature turned against Europe. No one is sure why the weather changed, but scientists studying tree rings and other data agree with old chronicles that it did change, and for the worse. The summer growing season became cooler and shorter. Rain fell longer and in heavier amounts. Glaciers in the Alps, having retreated for centuries, inched forward again, covering land used for grazing livestock. Ships once able to sail between Scandinavia and the Viking colonies in Iceland and Greenland found the seas blocked by ice.

Poor weather meant less food to go around—an ominous development, considering the European population had tripled over the previous three hundred years. There was no land left for expansion. Even the mediocre farmland was settled. To add to the crisis, many peasant farmers had exhausted the soil trying to grow more crops and keep up with payments to their landlords.

The average farmer's margin for error disappeared. Before, a bad year meant hardship. In the 1290s, and for decades thereafter, it spelled catastrophe.

And there were many bad years. Rain washed out the 1309 harvest across Europe. Abnormal amounts fell for the next decade. A bad harvest in 1315 was followed by a disastrous one in 1316. Famine struck Europe from England to Italy. Flooding caused by the rains led to outbreaks of water-related diseases like dysentery, typhoid, and malaria. All the ills related to malnutrition returned, as well. Even European livestock suffered epidemics—possibly rinderpest and anthrax—from 1316 onward.

Some scholars believe that the malnutrition and stress of the famine years led to long-term adverse health effects. That general weakening of Europe's health may have, years later, left its people vulnerable to the plague.

Europe was wet, hungry, sick, and demoralized. Asia, meanwhile, faced drought, then floods, then locust swarms—a litany of catastrophes capped by earthquakes that, according to one Chinese chronicle, caused an entire mountain to collapse.

The stress on the environment seems to have disturbed the rodent populations living on the steppe. Finding the changed conditions too harsh, the animals migrated into new habitats looking for food. The black rat was only one of the species on the move. Perhaps the most significant migrant was the marmot and its relative the tarabagan, another burrowing rodent hunted for its fur and as food.

The plague bacterium, living as it did in *X. cheopis*, traveled with the rodents. Once in a new place, the fleas hopped to the rodent species native to that habitat. Gerbils and jerboa caught it. So did rats and mice.

The affairs of rodents rarely concern human beings. But a change in human affairs began to steer humanity toward a collision with plague.

By the 1330s, merchant caravans had crisscrossed Asia for decades, protected by the so-called Mongol Peace. Before then, medieval peoples had seldom used the words "Mongol"

Plague-infested fleas also spread the disease to other rodent species like the marmot. Seen here in an 1882 illustration by Gustav Mützel is the bobak marmot, a species native to central Asia.

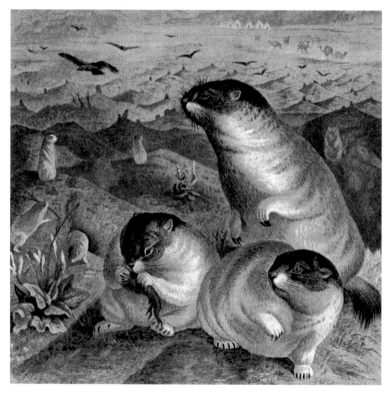

and "peace" in the same sentence. From the time Genghis Khan rode out of the steppe in the early thirteenth century, the Mongols were the terror of the medieval world. The Mongols earned their reputation through bloodthirsty conquest, but even their everyday habits revealed an almost unnatural toughness. According to European accounts, the Mongols tenderized meat by placing it under their saddles. The Mongols also believed that the dirt of human bodies corrupted rivers and other waters. Thus, they never bathed. Europeans—no great bathers themselves—considered them astonishingly filthy.

This Persian painting depicts Mongol warriors training for combat. The Mongol Peace of the 1330s allowed merchants to trade throughout Asia, facilitating the spread of diseases such as the plague.

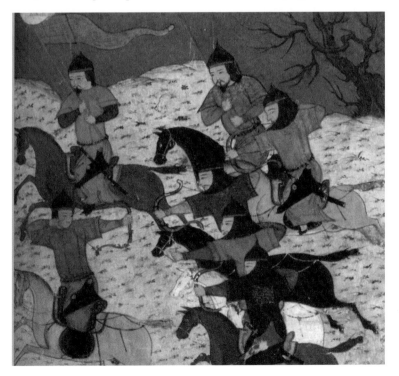

Having unified an empire that stretched from China to Russia, the Mongols created kingdoms (called khanates) and settled down to profit from their conquests. By enforcing the Mongol Peace, they freed merchants to travel across central Asia. Some of the roads went south to markets in India. Others connected Chinese cities to Europe and the Middle East. The Mongols, of course, profited from the trade.

The arduous eight- to twelve-month journey, made in relative safety (if considerable discomfort), promised a merchant profits and prestige. One of the popular routes took the caravans north, where the flat land was easier for carts and pack animals to navigate.

When a caravan made camp, the merchants and their workers came into contact with all kinds of curious and hungry local rodents. What made *Y. pestis* board the caravans cannot be known for certain. There are several possibilities. While *X. cheopis* prefers a rodent-blood meal, it has been known to feed on various other animals, and its tastes at the time may

The merchant caravans that traveled throughout Asia during the 1300s are believed to be responsible for the spread of the plague to Europe. *(Library of Congress)*

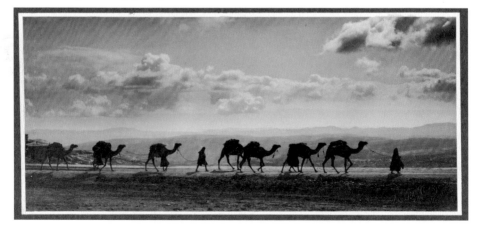

have included the blood of the camels used as pack animals by the caravans. It's also possible that a natural disaster of some sort had disrupted the local ecosystem, forcing the rodents to seek out the food stores of the caravan and bringing the rat fleas along for the ride. However it happened, rat fleas brought *Y. pestis* closer to human travelers. Eventually, the towns on the caravan routes began to suffer from plague.

Uncertain records make it hard to date the initial outbreak. The early or mid-1330s is an educated guess. Al-Mazriqi, an Egyptian historian, claimed the disease entered Persia from Mongol lands and left behind it a wasteland of death that spread all the way to Korea.

If that was the case, epidemics probably raged in Asia even as the Second Pandemic entered the West's historical record.

Lake Issyk Kul sits at over 5,200 feet above sea level in modern-day Kyrgyzstan. In the 1330s, a group of Christians belonging to the Nestorian sect lived in the area. Nestorianism was protected under the local khan's tolerant religious laws, and the community did well thanks to its proximity to the trade routes.

The evidence for plague among the Nestorians at Lake Issyk Kul is circumstantial, but weighty. While only four Nestorians died in an average year, gravestones in the community cemetery show more than one hundred people died in 1338 and 1339. In addition, the writing on some gravestones stated the deceased died of disease. That evidence, combined with the fact that marmots inhabited the local ecosystem, lead historians to believe that the Nestorians formed a link in the chain of infection as plague spread west.

In the early 1340s, those Europeans with an interest in foreign lands began to hear of terrible epidemics in the East. But

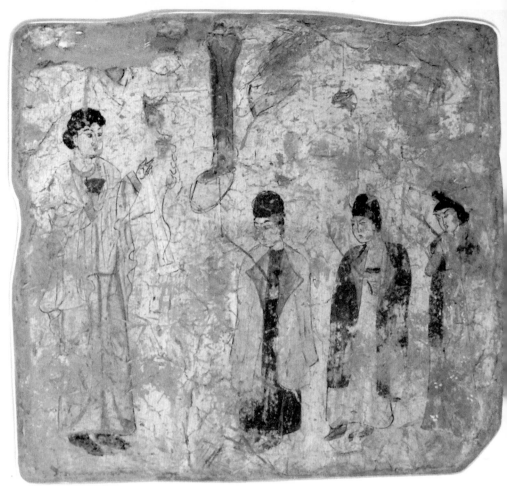

A wall painting of Nestorian priests. In 1338, a Nestorian sect in modern-day Kyrgyzstan became infected with the plague, forming a link in the chain of infection as plague spread west to Europe.

few people outside of the trading houses paid it much mind. Everyone knew strange things happened in exotic places like Cathay, as medieval Europeans called China.

Plague, meanwhile, came closer to Europe every year.

The khanate of the Golden Horde ruled "Great Sarai," and the city was the capital of a Mongol empire that covered much of central Asia and modern-day Russia. Goods brought to Sarai continued south, to where Italian traders kept fortified colonies on the Black Sea.

Genoa, one of the mightiest of the Italian trading states, had leased the city of Kaffa since 1266. From there, Italian galleys carried goods to European ports, at great profit to the Genoese. But Genoa's relationship with the Mongols was tense. First in 1343, and then again two years later, the Golden Horde attacked Kaffa. Though under siege on land, the Genoese fleet kept control of the Black Sea, an advantage they used to supply the city and bottle up the Mongol ships in their home ports.

Plague reached Sarai during the 1345 siege of Kaffa. The next year, it broke out in the Mongol armies surrounding the city. The epidemic was said to be devastating,

> . . . as though arrows were raining down from heaven to strike the Tartar's [Mongol's] arrogance. All medical advice and attention was useless, the Tartars died as soon as the signs of the disease appeared on their bodies: swellings in the armpit or groin caused by coagulating humors, followed by putrid fevers.

Gabriele de Mussi, an Italian notary, wrote those words in his account of the disaster. De Mussi was nowhere near Kaffa at the time. He lived in Piacenza, north of Genoa. Where he picked up the story is unknown, and it is unclear whether or not he ever spoke to merchants or sailors who witnessed the events. But if true, de Mussi's tale included a spectacular account of early biological warfare:

> The dying Tartars, stunned and stupefied by the immensity of disaster brought about by the disease, and realizing that they had no hope of escape, lost interest in the siege. But they ordered corpses to be placed in catapults and lobbed into the city in the hope that the intolerable stench would

kill everyone inside. What seemed like mountains of dead were thrown into the city.

In autumn 1347, ships carrying plague arrived at Alexandria, Egypt's major port. The Egyptian ruling caste imported horses, furs, and hides from central Asia. While *X. cheopis* will not live on horses, it could have traveled in the furs and hides or among the slaves the Egyptians also traded for.

The Islamic world was as stunned and stupefied as the Mongols. A thousand people died every day in Alexandria during the worst part of the epidemic. From there plague moved to Cairo, then throughout the Middle East. Damascus lost a quarter of its people. In Asyut, a Nile village, only 116 people paid taxes in 1349, down from 6,000 in previous years.

The Islamic world had known bubonic plague, albeit centuries before. The epidemics that followed Justinian's Plague continued in the Middle East and elsewhere for centuries, paralleling events in Europe. Plague had struck Syria roughly every ten years from Justinian's time until AD 745.

But the immensity of the new plague—what we know as the Black Death—surpassed the devastation of that earlier time. Bodies were stacked in streets because no room remained in the mosques. Alexandria ran out of coffins and burial shrouds. Authorities in urban areas dug trenches to dispose of bodies. Elsewhere, people left their dead on the roads or laid them out beneath trees.

The Black Death hit Tunis when the Arab historian Ibn Khaldun was a child. A later visitation would kill his parents. "The entire inhabited world changed," he said. "The East,

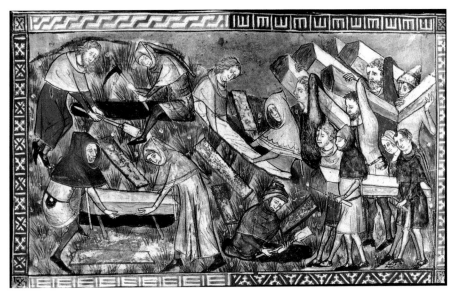

A 1349 illustration of plague victims being buried. *(Courtesy of The Granger Collection, New York/The Granger Collection)*

it seems, was similarly visited. . . . It was as if the voice of existence in the world had called out for oblivion and restriction, and the world responded to the call."

People turned to Islam to explain the disaster. In general, the Islamic faith made three pronouncements on epidemics:

- For Muslims, plague was martyrdom, and for non-Muslims, it was punishment;

- A land with plague should not be entered and those living in such a land should not leave;

- Plague came only from God, and therefore it could not possibly be contagious.

Each person decided the truth of these beliefs for himself. Many people, to be sure, either left plague-stricken regions, acted in ways to avoid contagion, or both.

It is possible a third of the Islamic world died, with death rates as high as 50 percent in the cities.

The Black Death, meanwhile, spread to continental Europe.

Merchant ships, possibly some originating in Kaffa, carried plague to Constantinople sometime in 1347. From there the disease went west with shipping. Due to the absence of advanced navigation, merchant vessels always sailed within sight of land rather than risking the open sea. Every few days the boats pulled into ports to resupply or sell goods. As Italian vessels made their way home, plague spread to coastal ports of call in Greece and the Balkans, and from those ports inland.

The Black Death arrived in Messina, Sicily, in late 1347. By January of 1348, it had made a spectacular landfall around the Adriatic ports, including Venice; in Genoa and several smaller Italian ports, all places connected by trade to Messina; and in Marseilles, the Mediterranean gateway to France. Some places were hit from two or more directions. That seems to have made the disease even deadlier.

Whereas Justinian's Plague did much of its damage in sea ports and adjacent areas, the Black Death traveled far into the countryside, even into remote regions. Throughout the spring and summer of 1348 it bored its way into the Italian interior. It whipped across southern France to English-controlled Bordeaux on the Atlantic Ocean, traveled via ship from continental Europe to Britain's southern coast, and followed river routes all the way to Paris.

Ships banned from Genoa and Marseilles arrived with it in Spain. Soon the disease spread tendrils across the entire Iberian peninsula—the Islamic kingdom of Grenada as well as the Christian lands of Castile and Aragon. Plague followed trade routes over the Alps into Switzerland and crossed the French frontier into the German-speaking lands of central Europe.

The next spring it raged with new lethality in Paris. As 1349 continued, the disease arrived in northern France and the Low Countries, slammed into Holland, crossed the North Sea from the British Isles to Norway. Soon it blazed in all Scandinavia. Ships again carried it to faraway lands, this time to Iceland and Greenland, the very edge of the European world.

The year 1350 saw plague dissipating in the lands where it first struck. But by then it had made its way to the borders of Russia, once again invading the lands of the Golden Horde and completing a circle of death around the continent.

The Black Death spread with extraordinary speed. In general, a pathogen advances slowly in a new disease pool. Progress tends to take place at a few miles per year. The Black Death spread several miles per day—it crossed France in only six months. After first striking Europe in 1347, the Black Death took roughly five years to spread from Constantinople to the tip of Spain and back again to the Russian interior. Even accounting for rats hitching rides on ships, it was an astonishing advance for an animal disease spread by an insect vector. Such pathogens tend to spread with animal populations, and animal populations, under normal circumstances, spread gradually.

No doubt the Black Death found conditions conducive to its spread. But its speed, as well as the ferocious death rates it inflicted, suggest the Black Death differed from Justinian's Plague in another important way.

The Black Death, in some places at least, was more than the noncontagious bubonic plague spread by fleas. Accounts

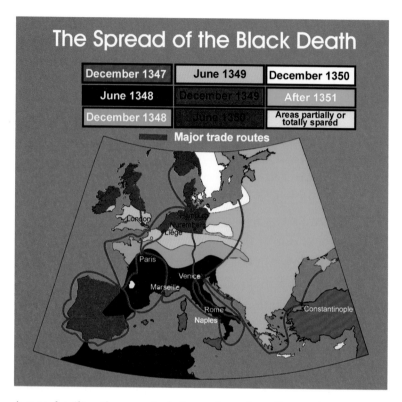

A map detailing the spread of plague throughout Europe from 1347 to 1357.

of the time claim it passed from person to person. That argues that the epidemic was, in part at least, the contagious pneumonic form.

The death rates associated with the Black Death underline the probability of pneumonic plague. Without treatment, and there was none in 1348, the pneumonic form kills close to 100 percent of the time. It also kills fast (as does the septicemic form). Accounts of the time agree that people died quickly. The Italian writer Giovanni Boccaccio made the dark-humored joke that one ate with one's friends at lunch and with one's ancestors at dinner. In addition, numerous medieval accounts often described both pneumonic symptoms and the despair of physicians and loved ones when victims began to cough up blood—a sure-fire sign the end was near.

The Black Death, in general, seems to have been a massive epidemic of both bubonic and pneumonic plague, with the blood-borne septicemic form a supporting player, and the shaky health of medieval people everywhere a major contributing factor.

One of the plague's enduring mysteries, however, is the evidence the Black Death acted in ways different than the plague studied in modern epidemics. The high death rates and the prevalence of the rare pneumonic form are but two of the differences. To take another, numerous observers in the Middle Ages said that plague patients gave off a terrible, corrupted odor. That is not seen—or smelled—in victims today and has yet to be explained.

Competing theories to explain the Black Death's behavior propose that it was a different strain of plague, that the plague of the time evolved in the 1330s to be contagious among human beings then burnt itself out, that the circumstances people lived under at that time played a complex role in plague's behavior but no longer exist today, or that an unusually deadly strain of "marmot plague" escaped from central Asia. A handful of scholars even claim the Black Death was not plague at all but another unknown disease.

To us, it is a set of mysteries to study. To the terrified people of the Middle Ages, however, it was an incomprehensible and very real catastrophe.

four
"The Dreadful Pestilence"

A person daring to go outside at the height of the Black Death stepped into a chamber of horrors. Black flags flew from the church steeple, warning outsiders that plague had come to the city. Lines of mourners tramped through narrow city streets bearing dead loved ones. Carts piled with corpses clattered by. Criminals and ex-slaves and the poorest workers dug immense pits to dispose of the bodies.

Dreadful noises came from the houses—sobs and curses of grief, the hungry cries of abandoned children, the prayers said for the living and the dead, the screams of bubonic plague victims in agonizing pain, and the thick coughs of those stricken with pneumonic plague.

Nobles, rich merchants, and priests deserting their parishioners clogged the roads, their carts packed with their valuables. The plague would travel with them to new regions—and new victims.

Those left behind prayed to St. Roch, the intercessor in plague cases, and sealed their drafty homes as best as possible. They did not know, and the science of the Middle Ages could not conceive, that fleas filled with a death-dealing bacteria had lived on the dead rats around their houses. As the rodents' bodies went cold, the fleas bounded through the cracks in the walls and dropped from the thatch roofs above—all searching for a warm-blooded host.

Nor did they know that the people in their neighborhood sneezed out a contagious and lethal form of the same disease carried by the fleas.

Death surrounded people, penetrated their hearts, and chilled their souls. The Italian poet Petrarch, like many people, lost numerous friends and loved ones to the disease, and he painted a vivid memory of what he had seen—a memory shared, in one form or another, by millions of his fellow human beings:

> Funerals meet my terrified eyes, wherever I turn them
> Horror piles upon horror, the churches crowded with coffins
> Echo to loud lamentations, while countless bodies unburied
> Noble and peasant alike, lie in the open unhonored.

The average European considered the Black Death the work of cosmic forces. Petrarch spoke to that, as well. "Either it is the wrath of God, for certainly I would think that our misdeeds deserve it, or it is just the harsh assault of the stars in their perpetually changing conjunctions. This plague-bearing year has borne down on humankind and threatens a tearful slaughter, and the highly charged air encourages death."

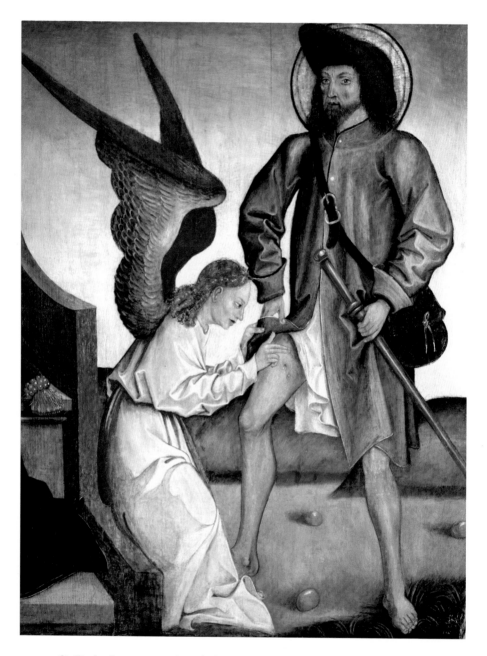

St. Roch, the patron saint of plague victims, being tended to by an angel. *(Courtesy of Interfoto Pressebildagentur/Alamy)*

Far more people connected the disease to God than to the stars. Even as the Black Death wracked cities and annihilated whole villages, priests thundered that Christians deserved it as punishment for their sins. Moralists celebrated the plague as proof of God's displeasure with all the offenses of the world—a displeasure they shared. The English writer Henry Knighton, for one, considered plague a "marvellous remedy" to outrageous women's fashions.

Not everyone agreed. Some Islamic scholars granted that the Black Death was God's will, but claimed it was also a natural disaster akin to a flood or earthquake. A number of European intellectuals agreed. Others looked at the misery and asked, If the plague is God's will, why did He punish the good *and* the wicked?

But even those inclined to disagree with the idea of divine punishment could not explain the Black Death with the science of the time.

The medieval doctor, ignorant of plague's causes and the manner of its spread, had no chance against it. The wiser practitioners recognized their limits. "Every pronounced case of plague is incurable," said Chalin de Vinario, one leading physician.

Doctors had far less status in the Middle Ages than they do now. In times of illness, people far more often visited one of the innumerable quacks, folk healers, and alchemists practicing at the time. Those sick in bed asked for the local priest. If a physician was called at all, he waited in the corner, a last-ditch option called upon only when prayer failed and the patient was near the end.

Medicine was hobbled by its loyalty to ancient ideas. Physicians still followed the teachings of the Roman doctor-

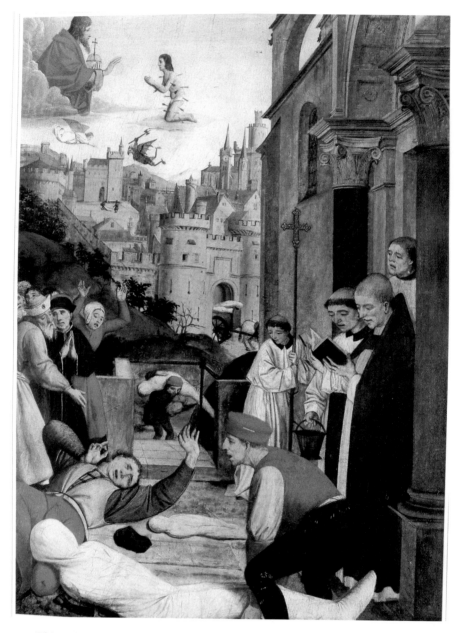

This 1497 painting shows plague sufferers begging for God's mercy outside a church as the dead collect in the streets. During this time, many believed the plague was proof of God's displeasure with humanity.

philosopher Galen (born c. AD 129). Galen had built on ideas inherited from the ancient Greeks and developed a complex system of medicine that endured—despite being wrong on almost every account—for 1500 years.

Galenic theory stated that good health depended on balancing the body's temperature and four humors: blood, phlegm (water), yellow bile, and black bile. For example, Galen advised bleeding patients who had a fever. Because he associated blood with heat, removing blood would, he said, cool the body. Bleeding with leeches (and other instruments)

Galen, a Roman doctor and philosopher, developed a complex system of medicine that endured for 1500 years. *(Courtesy of National Library of Medicine)*

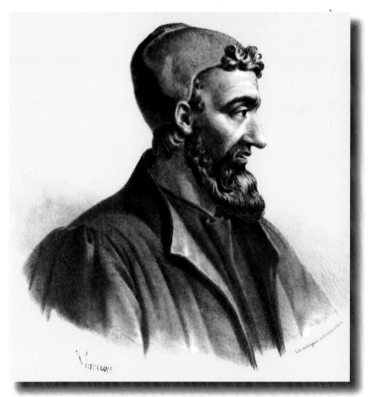

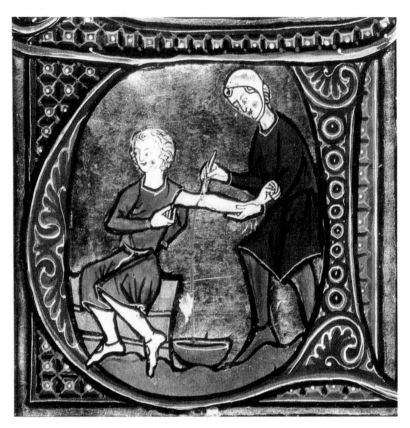

An illustration from the Middle Ages of a patient being bled. During this time, bleeding was a common medical practice based on Galen's theories about balancing the body's temperature and humors.

became a cure-all in ancient times and remained one in the Middle Ages.

Medical schools existed, but the education was limited. Students failed to learn much hands-on anatomy because Church law forbade the dissection of bodies for research or teaching. Instructors taught with pig corpses instead. To further confuse things, the Galenic medical texts in use were translations of translations of translations, and often incomplete besides.

Instead, astrology formed a significant part of a medical student's education. Hundreds of years before, Arab physicians had blended their complex astrological system with Galen and exported their ideas to Europe. There were medieval scholars who dismissed astrology as mumbo-jumbo. But it was hard to convince the physicians. After all, medical schools taught that casting a patient's horoscope was more important than a physical examination.

The average physician relied as much on common sense as anything else. In general, he took the attitude that, if God wished a patient to die, he could not hope to bring about a cure. It was his job to lend comfort. His orders to bleed a patient, the potions he prepared, and the advice he gave were not so much to cure as to keep the sick person psychologically strong. The patient went along with it or did not, depending on the individual.

Not surprisingly, doctors were not equipped to handle the Black Death. "The plague [was] shameful for the physicians," said the French physician Guy de Chauliac, "especially as, out of fear of infection, they hesitated to visit the sick."

Many fled town altogether. For years afterward, people held physicians in contempt for shirking their duty.

Terror of the plague unraveled friendships and undermined any sense of duty. Not only doctors ran away. When the Black Death arrived, the rich and powerful packed carts full of their prized possessions and got out of town: nobles and government officials, priests and physicians and wealthy merchants—one's position in society obviously meant nothing to the Black Death.

Saddest of all, terror of the plague often left a victim deserted by everyone, including his family. "The patient lay helpless and forsaken in his dwelling," said one account, "no relation came near him, at the most his best friends were huddled up in some corner. . . . With heart-rending supplication children called for their parents, parents for their children, the husband for the help of his wife."

Cities realized that the best way to deal with plague was to keep it out. As early as 1347, Genoa drove off suspicious "plague ships" with flaming arrows. (Disease nonetheless managed to enter the city at the end of the year.)

Venice was the first city to use quarantine. As Genoa's major rival, Venice carried on trade through the Black Sea and no doubt knew what had happened at Kaffa. Unlike most European cities of the time, Venice had a public health system, one led and staffed by professionals. The system provided the city with sanitation services and supported a system of

A view of Venice, Italy, the first city to employ quarantine methods to guard against the plague.

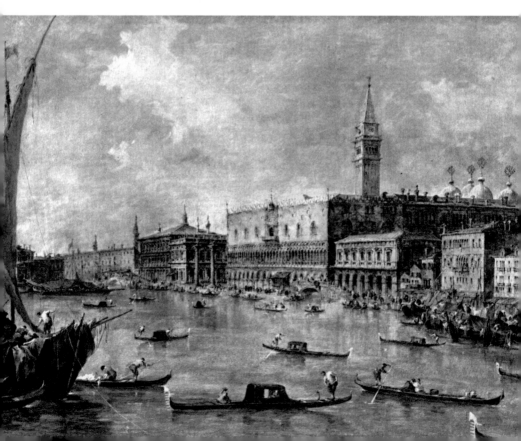

hospitals. With the Black Death on the move, the Venetian authorities enforced a quarantine on any suspicious ship. The quarantine lasted forty days—a period of time inspired by various Biblical events—and a ship's crew, along with its goods, waited it out on an island outside the city.

When plague got into Venice, officials turned to a strategy of isolating victims. By law, any plague case had to be reported. The sick were kept in their homes, as were those in recent contact with them. Guards were supposed to bring food and water to those inside, though in practice the guards abandoned them, out of apathy, drunkenness, or fear. The city buried the dead on islands and burned their clothes, linen, and other personal items.

Yet the Black Death hit Venice especially hard. Six in ten people may have died before the epidemic ended in mid-1349. In the aftermath, the city was so underpopulated that its leaders invited people from foreign lands to settle there, with a promise to accelerate the process for receiving citizenship.

It's possible, however, that similar public health measures worked elsewhere. Nuremberg, in southern Germany, had a sanitation system, banned the dumping of garbage on the streets, and supported public bathhouses. Many of the city's employers even included fees for bathing in their workers' pay. Whether these measures helped against plague, or whether the disease struck with less ferocity for other reasons, is uncertain. But Nuremberg had one of the lowest death tolls of any major European city.

Marseilles, the most important of France's southern ports, was one of Europe's wildest places. Its docks handled everything from spices to exotic animals to child slaves. Gangs roamed the streets. Even the monks got arrested for violent

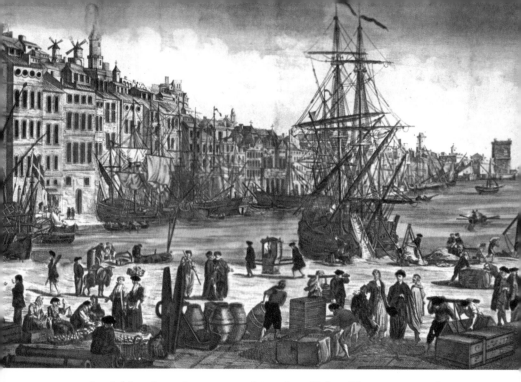

An eighteenth-century copperplate print of Marseille, a port town in France that became synonymous with the plague after an outbreak there in the fourteenth century.

crimes. From the time of plague's arrival in October 1347, the city became synonymous with the disease. Periodic outbreaks would continue until 1720, the last major epidemic in western Europe.

The Black Death unleashed in Marseilles what it unleashed in so many other places—streams of people fleeing in panic, corpses on the street and in houses and piled in carts, burial pits, chiming church bells, and mad prophets warning of God's anger and the end of the world.

But despite its lawless reputation, Marseilles maintained civic order. In fact, many of its citizens went about their business.

Documents from the period show that even as the Black Death raged, people negotiated business deals and got married. This practical response was actually common throughout Europe. Though one of history's worst disasters swirled around them, English farmers sewed their crops and Florentine lawyers wrote out the legal documents necessary to ensure smooth inheritances. Trade continued, if in reduced form.

Even war carried on. For years the Iberian peninsula had been the scene of civil wars and the ongoing conflict between Christian Castile and the Islamic Moors in the south. Alfonso XI of Castile was on the march again when the Black Death struck his Arab foes. Some of the Moors, impressed by the Christian God's power, thought about leaving Islam for Catholicism. Inevitably, however, plague broke out in Castile's ranks. Alfonso himself died of it on March 26, 1350.

Even as the plague spread throughout Europe and Asia, wars continued to rage. This fresco depicts Islamic Moors fighting in Spain in 1431.

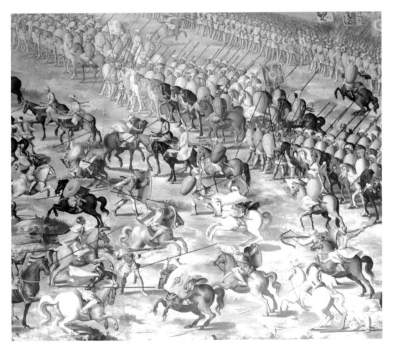

The plague's invasion of southern France threatened one of medieval Europe's few unifying institutions: the papacy. Due to complex political issues, Pope Clement VI lived at Avignon, north of Marseilles, rather than in Rome. The city was crowded with merchants, bankers, pilgrims, and Church bureaucrats, as well as business owners making money off all of them.

A nineteenth-century engraving of Pope Clement VI *(Courtesy of Roger Viollet Collection/Getty Images)*

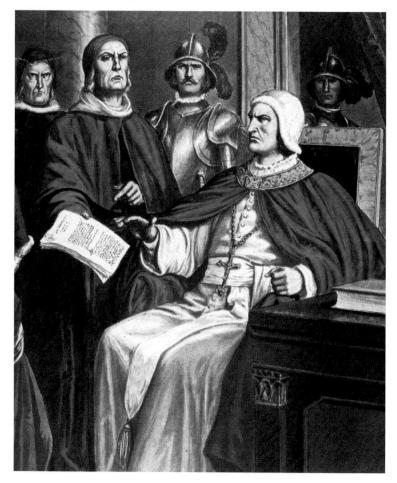

At the time, the Church was struggling with an image problem. Scandals and misbehavior had convinced a significant part of Europe that the clergy paid far more attention to making money and pursuing pleasure than to spiritual matters. (Pope Clement's enthusiasm for rich clothes, greyhound racing, and women did not help.)

The Black Death further undercut the Church's credibility. For one thing, the explanation that it was God's will sounded unsympathetic, if not offensive, to churchgoers mourning their loved ones. For another, the Church had no more control over the disease than anyone else, despite their claims to be God's representatives on Earth. In fact, plague killed priests, monks, nuns, and lay brothers at a terrible rate. But many others ran away. Respect for the Church and belief in its authority were two long-term casualties of the Black Death.

Avignon became a deadly place. Like other cities, it had trouble just disposing of the dead. The pope consecrated the local river so that Christians could be dumped into it. The monks at La Pignotte, an Avignon monastery, stayed to care for pneumonic plague victims. They paid for their show of mercy with their lives.

The Avignon physician Guy de Chauliac was one of the most famous doctors in Europe. Though respectful of the plague's power, he refused to run away, fearing it would give him a bad reputation. His description of the disease left no doubt both bubonic and pneumonic plague menaced Avignon:

> The mortality began with us in January and lasted for seven months. It had two phases. The first was for two months and with continuous fever and the spitting of

blood, from which victims died within three days. The second phase lasted for the remainder of the period and patients also had continuous fever. In addition . . . buboes . . . formed in the extremities, namely in the armpits and groin.

Chauliac was personal doctor to the pope and thus responsible for keeping Europe's spiritual leader alive. He advised Clement to sit between two raging fires in his quarters. Chauliac held the common belief that the smoke of the fires would overcome the "bad air" that infected people with plague. Clement survived the Black Death. While the smoke didn't keep him healthy, it did kill any fleas in his room. No doubt staying away from pneumonic townspeople also helped.

As the Black Death moved inland, communities went beyond quarantine in their efforts to escape. Tournai's town elders passed laws to stamp out sin. Couples living together were told to marry. New regulations prohibited playing dice or swearing. The German city of Speyer ordered citizens to cease gambling in the churchyard. In 1350, Magnus II, king of Sweden, told his subjects to walk to church barefoot and eat nothing on Friday except bread and water. He hoped (in vain) that the gestures would appease God's anger.

The survivors moved around in a haze of shock, fear, and grief. That people might give up, or even turn against their leaders, became a real threat—one authorities felt it essential to address before matters got out of hand.

With that in mind, lawmakers turned from punishing sin to keeping up morale. Many towns and cities forbade public mourning and ringing church bells at funerals, because so many people were in mourning and the bells rang all the time.

The elders in Pistoria, a town northwest of Florence, issued more specific rules. Mourners, with the exception of wives, were not to dress in new clothes. Paid mourners could not be hired for funerals. Nor could drummers. City fathers prohibited anyone from wailing over a person who died anywhere other than Pistoria.

Other reactions to the Black Death were more malevolent. Some people blamed it on the Jews.

The Jewish population had served as a scapegoat for European Christians for centuries. By a sad coincidence, several of the 1348 plague outbreaks occurred around Easter Week, a time of year when Christians went on anti-Jewish rampages. The two events dovetailed into acts of violence in France, the Low Countries, and particularly the German-speaking lands of Central Europe.

One of the first pogroms took place in Toulon, France, in spring 1348. Townspeople killed forty members of the Jewish community. The violence soon spread to other villages. In nearby La Baume, a mob burned the Jewish quarter.

Pope Clement ordered the persecution to stop, but the terror had already blossomed into widespread hysteria. As often happens in times of crisis, a conspiracy theory took shape. News of it spread as fast as the Black Death itself.

In simplest terms, the theory stated that Jews spread the plague on purpose in order to destroy Christianity. The belief gained strength in September 1348, when authorities arrested an unfortunate Jewish surgeon named Balavigny. When tortured—the French preferred the euphemism "put to the question"—Balavigny laid out a complex plot led by a mysterious "Rabbi Jacob" and orchestrated through a network of Jewish agents scattered across Europe.

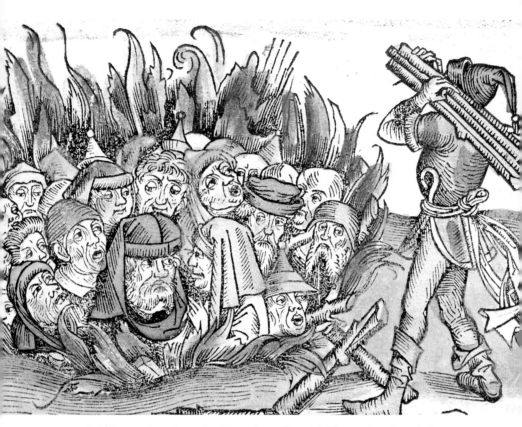

A 1493 woodcut from the *Nuremburg Chronicle* illustrating Jews being burned alive by those who believed them to be responsible for the Black Death.

The theory failed to stand up to logic. Plague killed Jews the same as it killed Christians, a point made by the pope himself. But, like many conspiracy theories, this one ran on prejudice and hysteria rather than reason.

From late 1348, and for months afterward, people attacked synagogues, burned the Jewish sections of towns and cities, murdered individuals, and butchered whole communities. The citizens of Basel pushed the entire Jewish population into a house and burned them alive. Brandenburg killed its Jews on a grill over a huge fire. Thousands of Jewish people died throughout the region between November of 1348 and August of 1349.

The pogroms often went hand-in-hand with another movement of the time. An event as apocalyptic as the Black Death, one so closely associated with God's wrath, led thousands to embrace religious fanaticism. The impulse had a colorful and dangerous outlet in the Flagellant movement.

Flagellant cults were nothing new. The Church had long used Christ's example to associate physical punishment with holiness. For decades prior to the Black Death, bands of men had traveled the roads putting on shows of self-torture in hopes that God would forgive their sins and those of others. Even in places where the authorities banned them, Flagellants appeared whenever disaster struck—whether it was a flood, a livestock disease, or the sight of a comet in the night sky. The Black Death, the disaster of all disasters, brought them out in greater numbers than ever before.

A 1349 illustration of a Flagellant procession

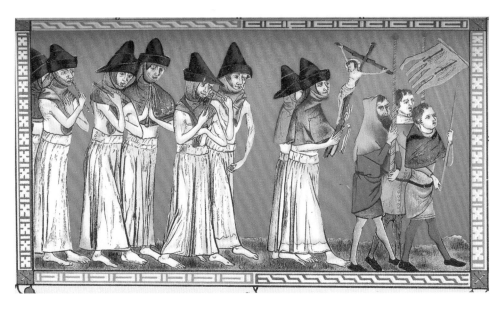

Groups like the Cross-Bearers and the Brotherhood of the Flagellants and the Brethren of the Cross were organized even as the epidemic was spreading. Each organization had a hierarchy—often supported by or including Church authorities—and a strict code of behavior.

Only a male could become a Flagellant. Before taking up duties, the would-be member had to confess all the sins he had committed since childhood. While on the march, the Flagellant pledged to whip his body three times a day, twice publicly and once privately. He also swore to be loyal to the leader of the band, called the Master or Father. Discipline was strict. Flagellants on the march could not wash or change clothes. They maintained silence except during rituals or when given permission to speak by the Master. Women, including Flagellants' wives, could not serve or speak to them. The length of a march varied but commonly lasted thirty-three-and-a-third days. (Christ had lived thirty-three-and-a-third years).

A Flagellant band arrived in a town to the sound of singing and church bells. Barefoot, dressed in hoods and white robes painted on either side with a red cross, the men trouped to the town church followed by singing and swaying locals.

Once at the church, the Flagellants stripped to the waist. To the horror and titillation of the crowd, the Flagellants marched in twos around the church, all the while whipping themselves. But this was only the first act. In sync, or sometimes one by one, the Flagellants fell to the ground. Each individual assumed the position of the cross or, in the case of severe sinners, a position that symbolized his worst sin.

As they lay there, the Master struck them gently with the knotted, spiked lash. The Flagellants then returned to their feet. They walked in a circle, lashing themselves in rhythm with accelerating ferocity, often trying to out-do one another, goaded by cries from the crowd. At certain points in their hymns they fell again to the ground, always praying, sometimes crying out in agony.

Finally, the Flagellants fell one last time. Locals rushed forward and, using rags or handkerchiefs, smeared Flagellant blood on their own cheeks.

Not content with their own performances, Flagellants provoked pogroms whenever possible. Supported by townspeople, they massacred Brussels's entire Jewish community and played a leading role in devastating others throughout Germany. Local authorities, even when opposed to the violence, often lacked the means to stop the mobs.

The Flagellant movement turned out to be short-lived. As time passed, the ranks were more and more filled by criminals and violent anti-Semites. More ambitious members, critical of the Church for a long time, saw a chance to damage it or seize some of its power and wealth for themselves.

Pope Clement condemned the movement, and his papal order had the force of law. Archbishops and bishops cracked down on clergy sympathetic to the Flagellants. Governments weary of the violence hunted down Flagellant bands and executed many of the members. The movement disappeared almost overnight. By autumn of 1350, less than two years after its initial appearance, the Flagellant hysteria had passed, to become a memory of a tragic interlude in a terrible time.

The Black Death struck England as the country was enjoying a recent upturn in its fortunes. Possibly in June 1348, and no later than August, plague broke out in several English ports. Henry Knighton wrote:

> Then the dreadful pestilence made its way along the coast by Southampton and reached Bristol, where almost the whole strength of the town perished, as it was surprised by sudden death; for few kept their beds more than two or three days, or even half a day. Then this cruel death spread on all sides, following the course of the sun.

Forty percent or more of Bristol's population may have died in a few months. The Black Death, meanwhile, traveled from the coast through southern England, a land of farms and small villages. It made its way to Ireland by ship and reached London, England's largest city, by the end of 1348.

London, like most medieval cities, was breathtakingly dirty. The lack of sanitation created an ideal home for black rats. That, combined with the constant assault on an individual's immune system by other urban diseases, made London—and for the same reasons Rome, Marseilles, Paris, and Amsterdam, to name just four—a perfect target for the Black Death.

Just an ordinary street scene was ghastly by modern standards. People emptied chamber pots of their body waste into the street, where it mingled with the piled droppings of local livestock. An animal that died in the street rotted wherever it fell. Surgeons dumped blood and other bodily fluids into gutters outside their shops. In theory, rainwater was supposed to wash the filth down gutters into rivers. Usually it washed it no more than a few blocks away.

The king at least had a pipe that carried the royal waste to a sewer. Nobles, lacking His Highness's resources, built their

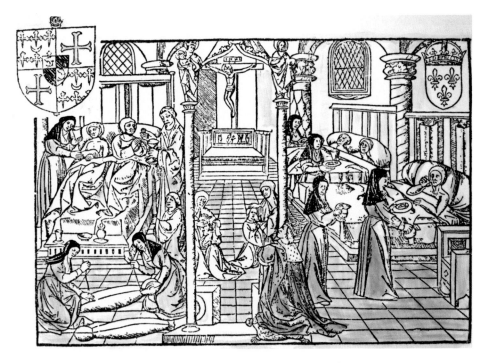

A 1490 illustration of plague victims in a Paris hospital *(Courtesy of Interfoto Pressebildagentur/Alamy)*

bathrooms over the Thames River or a ditch or let waste skid down their castle walls. Average Londoners resorted to tricks. In one famous case, two men steered their waste pipes into a neighbor's cellar.

Neither Londoners in particular nor Europeans in general helped their own cause. The average European seldom bathed—"seldom" being once a year, at best. Many never went into the water, never shaved, never changed their clothes. This aversion to cleanliness kept many of them covered in a mural of rashes and skin diseases. Head and body lice and the human flea *Pulex irritans* lived all over them.

It was small wonder, then, that the citizens of London—

and Avignon and Hamburg—struggled with any number of ailments before (and after) the Black Death arrived.

London may have suffered pneumonic plague in the cold months of 1348-49 and bubonic plague the following summer and autumn. What's known for certain is that the Black Death claimed many notable churchmen and government figures, in addition to masses of ordinary Londoners. Parliament declined to meet for fear of infection. Food became hard to find as farmers refused to enter the plague-stricken city. Famine was avoided only because the Black Death closed so many hungry mouths permanently.

The epidemic moved toward the North Sea, into the more isolated East Anglia region. As a wool-producing center, East Anglia received many ships from continental Europe. One or more brought the Black Death in the spring of 1349. Soon after, it arrived overland from London and other towns. Half of East Anglia's population perished—a death rate equal to some of the hardest-hit regions in all of Europe. Several villages became deserted and were never inhabited again. Surviving peasants migrated out of the area in numbers.

The Black Death's departure from Europe left behind it altered economies and weakened faith, the flame of new ideas and the smoking ruins left by old prejudices. People from China to Portugal, from the silent streets of Cairo to the empty farms of Viking Iceland, looked around at a changed world, in awe of the power of nature and the wrath of God.

five

The Long Aftermath and the Great Plague of London

The Black Death took an enormous toll on people's psychological, emotional, economic, and spiritual well-being. Countless human beings had lost loved ones and friends. Armies of orphans begged on city streets. We cannot know how many people never got over their grief or their anger at God or Allah, never returned to their previous place in society, or never found the strength to go on.

Writers of the time often noted, and just as often complained about, changes in behavior and attitudes. While each individual reacted to the plague in his or her own way, the changes that observers considered worthy of mentioning followed certain trends.

The people's opinion of the Church—mixed enough before the Black Death—fell further. The clergymen who had fled from the plague to save their lives eclipsed the selfless actions of those who stayed behind to care for the sick. A church-man walking the streets of post-plague Europe blushed at the insults thrown his way.

Even Pope Clement had harsh words for his priests. "[A]bout what can you preach to the people?" he declared. "If on humility, you yourselves are the proudest of the world, arrogant and given to pomp. If on poverty, you are the most grasping and most covetous. . . . If on chastity—but we will be silent on this, for God knoweth what each man does and how many of you satisfy your lusts."

There was also a spike in the crime rate. Crime had, in fact, never stopped, not even during the epidemic's darkest days. One notorious Englishwoman, Catherine Bugsey, spent the Black Death stealing clothes from dead bodies. (She never caught plague.) Gangs of grave-diggers, former slaves called *becchini*, terrorized Florence. Empowered to enter plague victims' houses, the *becchini* went anywhere they wished, forcing bribes from sick people, dragging the well to isolation houses if they refused to pay, and committing every kind of crime. Nor did plague deter white-collar crime. Officials in Florence skimmed a fortune in gold from the estates of plague victims.

Legal sinning rose, as well. "Men . . . gave themselves over to the most disordered and sordid behavior," said the Italian writer Matteo Villani. "As they wallowed in idleness, their dissolution led them into the sin of gluttony, into banquets, taverns, delicate foods and gambling. They rushed headlong into lust."

There seemed no end to it. Survivors lived together outside of marriage in great numbers, many of them no doubt wid-owed survivors of the Black Death. Those with a little money

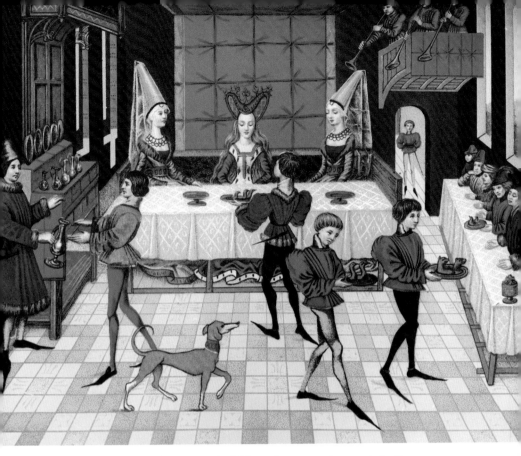

This illustration shows a typical fifteenth-century banquet. In the years following the Black Death, the population began to indulge more and celebrate life. *(Courtesy of Lebrecht Music and Arts Photo Library/Alamy)*

preferred to block out the worries of the world and retreated into enjoyment of the best food, hearty wine, and evenings spent in charming conversation.

Changes in fashion were especially scandalous. The strict dress codes for women before the plague gave way to low-necked tops and luxurious wigs. Men did their part by choosing to wear short coats, the forerunner of today's jacket. The coats, and in fact various clothes for both sexes, hugged the body, revealing contours that offended their conservative neighbors. Bright colors became fashionable, as did pointed shoes. Peasants and artisans even dared to drape themselves in furs, as if they were lords. King Edward III of England felt moved to pass laws against such impertinence. Dutch textile makers, famous for their drab but functional clothes, took a sharp loss of business.

The changes represented more than a newfound love of life. The Black Death had reshuffled society's cards. The survivors had more money. Just as importantly, workers could demand better pay because so few of them were left alive. Rural landlords scrambled to find people to harvest wheat or graze sheep. The peasants demanded more pay, fewer taxes, and better treatment. If refused, they left to take one of the plentiful jobs available elsewhere. At the same time, urban workers asked for and got higher wages—high enough to buy pointy shoes, even.

All of the playfulness and independence, however, masked a widespread feeling of grim fatalism. The Black Death had seemed to come from nowhere. What even greater disaster would be next? Europeans lived their lives in a state of constant strain. Every heavy rainfall inspired someone to predict floods or famine. Priests, believing the end of the world must be near, used their Sunday sermons to warn that the Antichrist walked the earth.

And then plague returned. It would thereafter remain a part of European life, and a prolific killer, for more than three hundred years.

Europeans called it the *pestis secundus*, Latin for second plague. It arrived in western Europe in 1361 and killed a fifth of England's remaining population. There were similar losses on the continent—in some places, the dying exceeded that of the Black Death. As if plague weren't enough, several countries had to deal with a simultaneous epidemic of smallpox.

Plague changed its behavior as it became a part of Europe's ecosystem. Pneumonic plague, probably frequent during the Black Death, became rare again. Septicemic plague remained so. The bubonic form dominated, with rats and the flea vector primarily responsible for the outbreaks in 1361 and thereafter. Epidemics returned in cycles every six to twelve years, but the disease circulated among the poor the rest of the time, picking off a few people here and there every year. Outbreaks usually happened in the summer, unlike the year-round horror of the Black Death. Most struck on a local scale, a city or a region, rather than countrywide.

Port cities remained the most vulnerable. Each dealt with its own local plague. But occasionally a ship brought in a more virulent strain from the Middle East or western Asia. When that happened, severe plague broke out in places like Venice and Marseilles, with deaths in the thousands.

Plague remained a mystery to the medical profession, despite its frequent presence. Physicians were baffled by its habits and unable to fit it into Galen's theories. But that did not stop experts from coming up with an extensive lore of preventatives and cures.

The Islamic scholar Ibn Khatimah wrote widely on the subject. His advice was typical Galenic medicine. For instance, he put great stock in keeping the body cool and quiet. Bleeding to remove "hot" blood was a must. The sun and objects like ovens had to be avoided. He cautioned against exercise, as well. Physical exertion heated up the body, and hurried breathing brought more infected "bad air" into one's body. It also opened the pores, an invitation to infections.People had associated disease with bad odors since ancient times. Of particular danger, however, was miasma, an odious substance

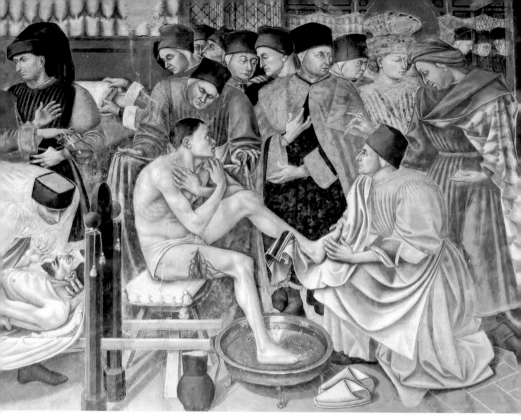

A fifteenth-century painting of patients surrounded by physicians. Although the plague was a common illness at the time, medieval physicians lacked the medical knowledge to prevent or treat the disease.

(or foul-smelling fog) generated in nature. The Greeks believed swamps emitted miasma, a view adopted by Galen and the Romans. By the Middle Ages, European and Arab intellectuals had expanded the theory. It was said that miasma could also form over open water and creep ashore as a deadly mist. Ibn Khatimah believed the rays of the sun and stars encouraged miasma by adding dangerous warmth and dampness to the air.

Physicians suggested a person surround himself with pleasant smells to offset dangerous odors. The English and the Dutch considered strong-smelling tobacco essential to good health. By the 1600s, students at one English boarding school had to smoke every morning or be flogged.

Both European and Islamic experts advised burning woods with strong scents. Ash, juniper, and cypress were favorites. Herbs like thyme and mint were also acceptable, as were aromatic oils. Burning sulfur was one of the less-pleasing recommendations.

One authority told urban readers to surround their towns with sweet-smelling shrubbery. People able to afford it spread flowers on their beds. Rubbing violets on the body (or drinking a violet tea) persisted as a remedy in Egypt into the 1700s. Ibn Khatimah advised sprinkling a rosewater-vinegar mixture around the house and rubbing one's face with lemon or flowers like roses and violets. None of this prevented plague. But it did improve the smell of people's houses.

Doctors in plague-ridden Marseilles developed tools along these lines. By the 1600s, physicians in the city wore masks shaped like beaks. The beaks were stuffed with spices and herbs that supposedly filtered out the plague-carrying odors.

Another widespread remedy was the smelling apple, a hand-held container of spices, flowers, and other scents held near the nose as one walked around. Recipes for smelling apples varied but might include ingredients like roses or black pepper.

An opposing theory stated that unpleasant odors acted as a sort of vaccine. Hospital workers, gravediggers, butchers, and others surrounded by vile smells were said to be immune to plague. This led to scenes of proper upper-class citizens bent over latrines for hours to fight fire—plague—with fire—strong odors.

Diet, too, was believed to be an important part of plague prevention. Unfortunately for those needing good advice, the experts rarely agreed with one another.

A seventeenth-century illustration of a physician wearing a plague prevention mask. Plague was thought to be caused by bad odors, so doctors wore masks filled with spices and herbs that supposedly filtered out the dangerous smells. (*Courtesy of Wellcome Library, London*)

Some Arab doctors advised eating one pickled onion a day to keep plague away. Ibn Khatimah, however, told patients to avoid fragrant foods, as well as heavy meals like oatmeal and cheese. Better to eat fruit, he said—plums and white grapes especially—and drink fruit juice. Bread was also desirable, the coarser the better.

Instructors at the Paris medical school—considered to be the foremost experts on such matters—said to avoid lettuce. Others, however, advised cool leafy vegetables. Many sources agreed that foods prone to spoiling, like meat and milk, were bad. Ibn Khatimah allowed eggs, but only those dipped in vinegar.

One of the stranger cures was actually quite popular. Galen had instructed his patients to devour red Armenian clay, which was red due to its iron oxide content. Ibn Khatimah believed in the clay's healing power, as did Guy de Chauliac. Other physicians packed the healing clay around a victim's buboes.

As with modern health care, psychology played an important part in healing. Everyone agreed that a calm and happy state of mind was a powerful preventative. Negative emotions, on the other hand, left one vulnerable. The German doctor Jobus Lincelius said:

> Physical exertions and emotions of the mind should be avoided, such as running, jumping, jealousy, anger, hatred, sadness, horror or fear, licentiousness and the like, and those who, by the grace of God, are in a position to do so, may spend their time in relating tales . . . and with good music to delight their hearts. . . .

Ibn Khatimah warned that the mental energy associated with intelligence was a risk. When it came to infection, stupidity was a more desirable state of mind. Many experts advised a modest intake of wine, but just enough to improve the mood without bringing on drunkenness.

Science progressed throughout the Renaissance and the centuries that followed, but magic remained an important part of everyday life in the years of the Second Pandemic. The unpredictability of plague made it seem like a supernatural event, all the more so since no one understood how the disease worked or spread. Fake doctors, false holy men, astrologers, potion brewers, and old women sold a bewildering variety of preventatives to the desperate and gullible. Real physicians, having few real cures, often got into the business themselves.

Snakes, with their connection to poison, played an important part in healing lore across Europe and the Islamic world. Ground-up snake parts went into many potions. On at least one occasion people wore the tongues of venomous species on their bodies to protect against disease.

Victims soaked their buboes in egg yolks or covered them with dead toads dried according to specific rules. Italians had used the enchanted word *abracadabra* against malaria since ancient times. It was adapted into a charm against plague, too. The famed Italian physician Gentile de Foligno considered powdered emerald a peerless—if expensive—cure for disease. In Poland and Prussia, people ate pieces of buboes in their food or in some cases swallowed pus taken from victims.

Magical remedies often went hand-in-hand with religious faith. Devout Muslims printed the opening words of the Quran inside cups and bowls, then poured in water to dissolve the print. The inky water would, it was thought, protect against plague if consumed or poured into bath water. Preachers in

Krakow, Poland, sold magic coins bearing the picture of St. George. Con men, meanwhile, sold amulets that supposedly contained scrolls written by saints or by the Virgin Mary.

The lack of knowledge about plague did not prevent governments from tackling the problem. Cities like Florence and Venice kept a staff of full-time medical specialists to identify and act against outbreaks of disease. Professional health boards kept track of records and maintained quarantine houses—called lazarettos, or pesthouses—to isolate the sick. Authorities continued to quarantine ships.

Knowledge, however, had yet to catch up with human need. The lazarettos were not so much hospitals as places to imprison the sick. The filth inside actually encouraged disease. Attendants mistreated victims or ignored them. Patients mad with pain or fever wandered the halls screaming. During epidemics, corpses piled up. People so dreaded pesthouses

An etching of a lazaretto in Italy. Although lazarettos were meant to be hospitals for plague victims, most became prisons for the sick. *(Courtesy of Wellcome Library, London)*

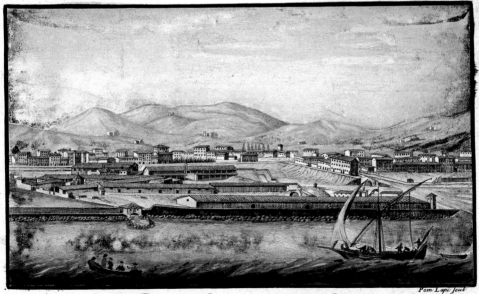

Veduta del Lazzeretto di S: Rocco

that they sometimes killed themselves rather than be sent to one.

Authorities took preventative measures into citizens' homes. In 1630, as plague raged in Florence, the government confiscated mattresses—said to harbor miasma—and burned them. The city replaced the bedding at its own expense. Spain had done the same at the beginning of the century and torched linen and clothes, too.

Wave after wave of bubonic plague nonetheless returned into the 1600s. Three outbreaks in Spain between 1596 and 1685 may have killed 1.5 million people and contributed to the decline of the Spanish Empire. But the best-known epidemic of the era, the Great Plague of London, struck England in 1665.

From the mid-1650s on, plague was on the move again across vast spaces. In 1654 it hit Moscow, then returned to Naples and Genoa by the end of the decade. England remained clear as late as 1663, but all of Europe knew that bubonic plague had re-entered port cities in Holland and Germany, in Scandinavia, and around the Baltic Sea. All carried on a heavy trade with the English, particularly in cloth and timber.

It was a time of omens. On November 18, 1664, a spectacular comet appeared. Isaac Newton studied its progress through the following January; King Charles II and his queen observed it on December 17. Comets, as everyone knew, preceded disaster. The personal astrologer of Czar Alexei of Russia warned of pestilence and catastrophe.

The comet arrived as King Charles II planned war against Holland. Impending hostilities did not prevent a thriving English-Dutch trade. War was war, but business was business. With plague infecting Holland's ports, however, trade—

much of it in cloth—risked spreading the epidemic to English ports.

Charles had recognized the danger. A year before, he ordered Dutch ships from stricken cities to be quarantined. But the regulations were hardly airtight. Dutch officers jumped ship to visit friends or relatives in England, while government officials, the king included, waived the quarantine for naval supplies or other special purchases.

A country so interconnected with the outside world could not hold out forever. In late 1664, as the comet flared in the night sky, bubonic plague broke out in London.

It started in the poor suburban areas (called "liberties") outside the city walls. Then the daughter of a doctor died of plague in Westminster, the town west of London where the king and other wealthy citizens made their homes. Officials reacted by covering up the news. It took until the last week of April for the government to admit a crisis. By then, bubonic plague had broken out in St. Giles in the Fields, a poverty-stricken area north of Westminster.

Unlike Venice, London did not pay much attention to public health. In Venice, trained professionals evaluated the sick or the dead to determine if plague was present. London depended on old women who scooted from house to house and might give any diagnosis for a price. Nor did the city maintain pesthouses. It was the English habit to throw quarantine buildings together with each new epidemic. Officials instead ordered houses with plague to be boarded up, with all inhabitants—sick or well—inside. When the government attempted that in 1665, residents in St. Giles in the Fields replied to the order with rioting. Those in other areas resisted similar regulations.

Plague spread, first to the nearby liberties and then to London itself. As in the past, many of those able to flee did so. But most Londoners, having no choice, remained. The artisans and workers, the apprentices and jobless poor, could not afford to quit working, let alone pack up and leave the city.

Samuel Pepys, though not a poor man, decided to stay. Ambitious and life-loving, Pepys made his living acquiring goods for the British Navy. With England locked in a naval war with Holland, a driven businessman like

This wood engraving depicts a street scene in London during the 1665 plague outbreak. *(Courtesy of Wellcome Library, London)*

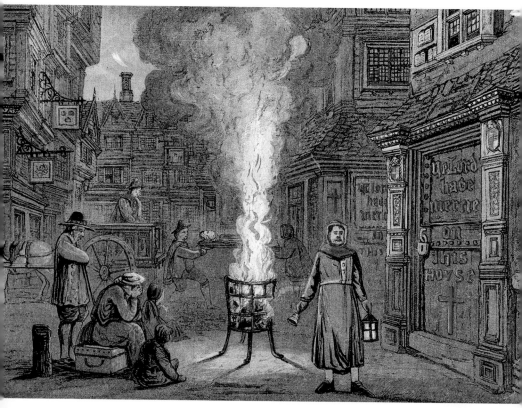

Pepys considered it worth risking plague to chase wartime profits.

As he hurried through the streets, Pepys heard the incessant ringing of church bells in London and the liberties. He passed large bonfires started in order to cleanse the airs of miasma, noted the rising death count in published government documents, and saw boats dotting the Thames River as thousands of people hoped to ride out the plague on water.

Schools closed, as did the courts. Pepys complained about the ban on theaters; other Londoners believed the closing of taverns and inns too extreme. Church services were allowed, but only those of the official Anglican Church. Quakers, Jews, and members of other religious groups went to prison if they dared to meet.

But still the epidemic grew. The government reported 2,815 plague fatalities the first week of August. By the week of August 22nd to 29th , the death count had almost tripled. On the last day of the month Pepys wrote:

> Thus this month ends, with great sadness upon the publick through the greatness of the plague everywhere through the kingdom almost. Every day sadder and sadder news of its encrease. In the City died this week 7,496 and of them 6,102 of the plague. But it is feared that the true number of the dead, this week is near 10,000[.]

The official figure climbed to just short of 7,000 the next week. The unofficial but truer figure, counting poor people and others hard to trace, was far higher.

But Pepys' diary shows that during the Great Plague, as during the Black Death, some Londoners attempted to continue with their everyday lives. In mid-September, for example, with the epidemic at its peak, Pepys worked on side deals for silk and cinnamon, worried over his financial books, and skirted a scandal involving luxury goods seized from the Dutch.

By autumn, plague was, as Pepys had written, everywhere in the kingdom almost. Fleeing Londoners helped spread it across the south. Others making their way to Colchester found the disease waiting for them in rural villages. In fact, it had already reached Colchester, possibly via *X. cheopis* hiding in cloth shipments. Half of that city's 10,000 people would die.

Similar circumstances brought plague to Eyam, a village located in the middle of England.

Eyam's experience became one of the famous stories of the time. In September of 1665, a shipment of cloth arrived from London for the village tailor. The tailor died of bubonic plague a few days later. The disease spread, and the townspeople prepared to flee.

But William Mompesson, the local rector, convinced them they should stay. To leave, he said, would spread plague to other parts of the kingdom, perhaps across the whole north of England. The town agreed. The sacrifice may have saved many of the region's villages and towns. But Eyam suffered huge losses. The disease lingered late into the next year. Of the 350 villagers, 260 died of plague, Mompesson's family among them.

In London, the number of plague cases began to decline in October, though the disease lingered well into the next summer. At the end of 1665, the government listed the plague dead at 68,596. Historians, aware the figure missed many of the poor, accept that at least 100,000 people perished.

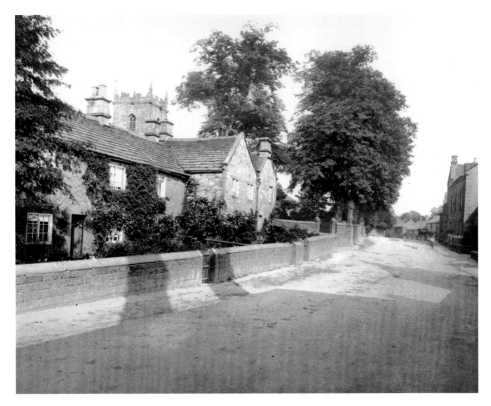

Eyam, the English village where residents quarantined themselves to keep the plague from spreading. *(Library of Congress)*

Pepys wrote on December 31, "My whole family hath been well all this while, and all my friends I know of, saving my aunt Bell, who is dead, and some children of my [Cousin] Sarah's, of the plague. But many of such as I know very well, dead. Yet to our great joy, the town fills apace, and shops begin to open again."

One more disaster awaited London. In September of 1666, a fire started in a bakery. Much of the city burned. For a long time it was believed the fire put an end to the plague. That was untrue. But the city did make improvements that helped

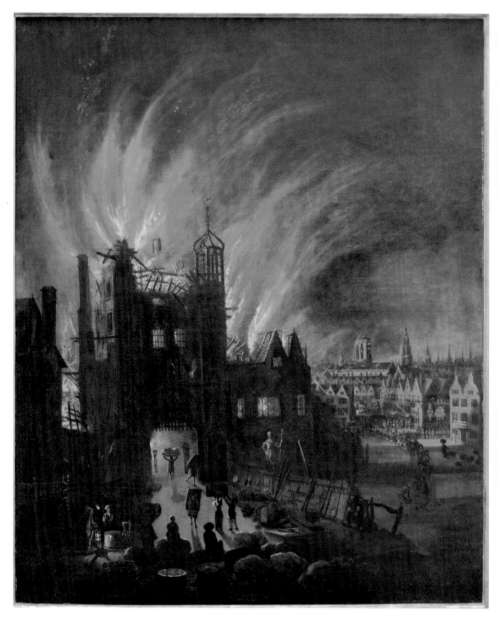

A painting of St. Paul's Cathedral during the London fire of 1666

prevent later outbreaks. Londoners rebuilt the city using stone and brick instead of rodent-friendly wood. Thatch roofs disappeared, replaced by tile. The rats and fleas, left homeless by the changes, moved outdoors, away from human beings. The Great Plague of 1665-1666 marked London's last major epidemic.

But the Second Pandemic continued elsewhere.

The last major outbreak in western Europe took place in 1720, at Marseilles, when ships brought a ferocious plague from the east. Russia and eastern Europe continued to be hit by epidemics throughout the 1700s. Another great plague struck Moscow more than a century after the London epidemic.

In the 1740s, Russian colonists were migrating into the steppe regions in the southern part of the empire. Hundreds of years before, caravans carrying goods and plague from Asia had crisscrossed the region. War, epidemics, and migration had since left the region mostly deserted—by humans, anyway. Vast rodent colonies still honeycombed the steppe's fertile soil. The rats and gerbils still hosted *X. cheopis*. And the plague flea still infected local rodents with *Y. pestis*.

Moscow, one of Russia's major cities, was vulnerable to plague for many reasons. It had the problems of filth and poverty and poor housing common to all cities. It was also a clearinghouse for grain, a favorite rat food, and the city's wooden houses, as usual, made excellent rat homes. To add to the threat, the tough Norway (or gray) rat had joined the black rat, giving the city two efficient plague carriers.

In 1770, Russia's army was at war with the Ottoman Turks. Soldiers on the move spread bubonic plague, as did traders and refugees. The disease arrived in Kiev, in the Ukraine, in late August. By October, it had spread through the rodent

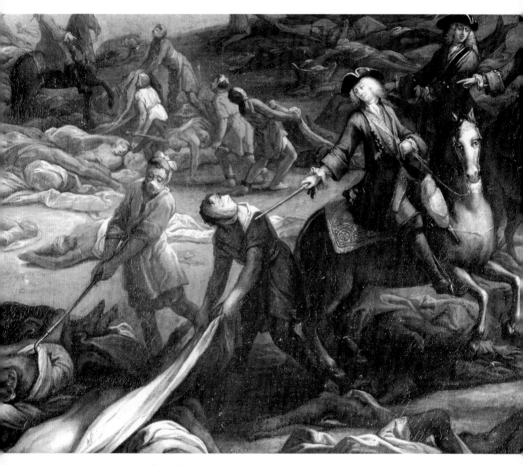

A painting of workers clearing the dead from the streets of Marseille during the last great plague outbreak there in 1720. *(Courtesy of Getty Images)*

population and was exploding among the humans. The empress, Catherine the Great, ordered Kiev sealed off.

But it was to no effect. For weeks, plague crept toward Moscow despite quarantines, inspections, and the burning of suspect goods. It probably arrived in the city in early November of 1770. As had happened in Justinian's Plague and the Great Plague of London, the initial cases were modest in number, and though doctors feared an epidemic, the threat of disease abated as cold weather set in.

And, as in those other locales, plague returned the next year. An epidemic built up through the spring and early summer of 1771. Peasants working with Persian and Ottoman fabric in the textile factories began to die. By September, Moscow was in the grip of an epidemic. Panic turned to riots, and the riots turned into a street battle between locals and the authorities.

One Russian merchant wrote:

> The [common] people began to scatter to nearby towns and villages and some of them were themselves already infected, while others carried off clothing and other things impregnated with that death-dealing poison, so the infection multiplied among many towns and villages, and especially the villages that lie close to Moscow lost more than half their inhabitants.

Plague killed 52,000 people, possibly more, in Moscow. At least 75,000 died in the rest of the Russian Empire.

For Europe, at least, the Second Pandemic was coming to an end. But plague did not vanish from the world. Rodents continued to die of it, as they had for so long, in Manchuria and central Asia. The disease also took the odd marmot hunter, villager, or other poor soul unlucky enough to come into contact with *Y. pestis*. Occasional larger outbreaks shook Russia's Black Sea area, the Middle East, and parts of north-central Africa.

Only a hundred years after the Moscow epidemic, a third pandemic took shape in the Chinese interior. Its point of origin would be as mysterious as that of the preceding pandemics. But this time the plague would travel faster and it would travel farther, to Pacific islands and the crowded streets of India—in fact, to every settled continent on Earth.

six

The Current Pandemic

The Third Pandemic of plague, and the one currently in progress, began in the 1860s in Yunnan, a region of southwestern China. The epidemic soon traveled a thousand miles east to Pakhoi. After outbreaks there in 1877 and 1882, it killed 70,000 in Canton.

In 1894, bubonic plague arrived in Hong Kong. From that British colony, *Y. pestis* would extend its reach around the world.

The plague first took root in the city's poor areas, where giant port rats prowled the alleys and human immune systems faltered in the face of unsanitary living conditions, overwork, and bad food. At first, the British colonial authorities in charge in Hong Kong refused to believe the disease on the loose there was bubonic plague. That the reports concerned poor Chinese made them less-than-convincing, too. Condescending British citizens sniffed that all kinds of diseases circulated among

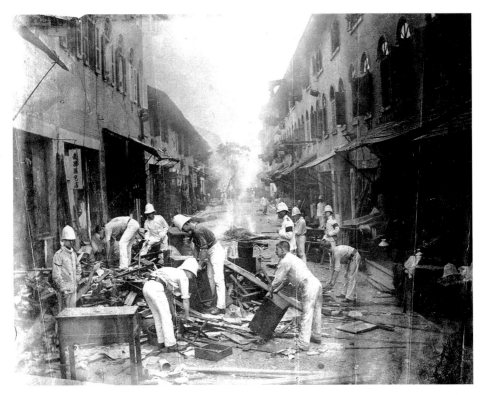

An 1894 photo of British troops cleaning out plague houses in Hong Kong. *(Courtesy of Wellcome Library, London)*

"those people." How could anyone tell bubonic plague from the others?

Whatever happened in a busy port like Hong Kong soon reached the outside world. Reports of plague, denied or not, created a sensation—and fear.

But much had changed since the dire epidemics of the past. As the Third Pandemic began, science was equipping humanity with the knowledge to fight back against the disease.

The late nineteenth century was a time of enormous scientific advance. Few if any fields came so far so fast as biology in general and medicine in particular. Assisted by breakthroughs in related technology like microscopes, and using observation and experimentation to establish scientific proofs, researchers like Louis Pasteur and Robert Koch had spearheaded a revolution. Knowledge of human pathogens increased more in a few decades than in the previous thousand years combined. Pasteur's and Koch's investigations, and those of other scientists using their methods, opened up a new era of disease prevention that led to similar advances in the treatment of infectious disease.

Until the 1890s, however, plague was left uninvestigated, in large part because the sweeping epidemics of the past were

Louis Pasteur

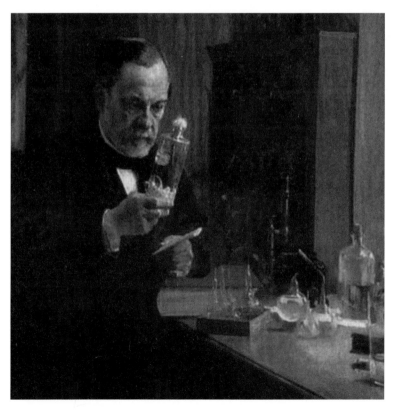

considered more a matter of history than science. The Hong Kong outbreak changed that perspective. Here was the terrible killer of the Middle Ages, back in the modern day. The scientific community recognized Hong Kong's problem as a historic opportunity to study bubonic plague as it happened, to find out what caused it and where it came from.

When the British governor of Hong Kong sent an international plea for help, no less a scientist than Shibasaburo Kitasato responded.

Shibasaburo Kitasato *(Courtesy of Wellcome Library, London)*

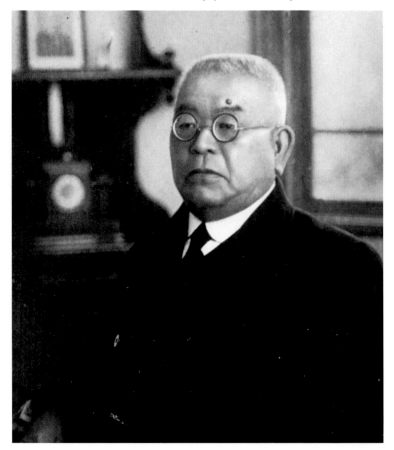

Kitasato had made his name from his groundbreaking work on the tetanus bacterium, a major cause of human infection. The taciturn, stout Japanese scientist was considered one of the world's foremost bacteriologists, and the British authorities were thrilled to have his help. He arrived the second week of June 1894, and received every courtesy from his hosts: dinners with the medical services director, the nickname "The Professor," and most important of all, space to set up a laboratory for himself and his staff of experts and assistants.

Kitasato went to work immediately. Barely twenty-four hours after the Japanese team arrived, he believed he had found the plague bacterium. Kitasato sent the news to the *Lancet,* the world's foremost medical journal. Word that he had unlocked plague buzzed through the scientific community and made its way into the press.

The problem was, he had actually found something else.

Kitasato's mistake opened the door for a second researcher, Alexander Yersin. Yersin had lived the life of a character in an adventure novel. After starting and then giving up a brilliant career in science, Yersin journeyed to Indochina, France's colony in Southeast Asia, to work as a doctor. He was a far more enthusiastic explorer. Living on rice, making detailed maps, sympathetic to the Indochinese, Yersin trekked throughout the region for much of the early 1890s and was the first European to see many areas of the interior. Along the way he faced down bandits and fled angry villagers who were convinced that a man with white skin had to be a witch.

Yersin had for some time asked his bosses for permission to study plague in southern China. When he heard news of the Hong Kong outbreak, he used his connections to get sent

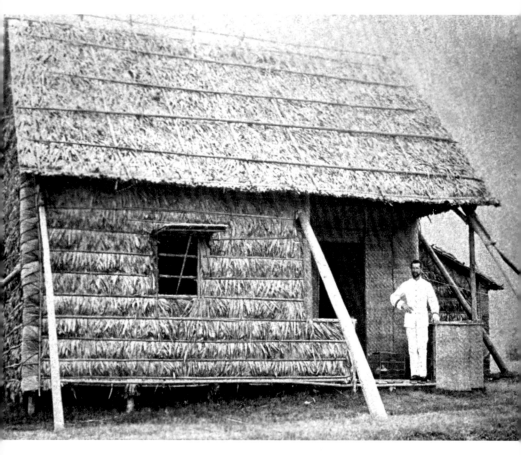

Dr. Alexander Yersin in front of the straw laboratory building where he first isolated and identified the bacteria that causes plague. *(Courtesy of HKU-Pasteur Research Centre)*

to the city. He left with a few suitcases of equipment and two assistants.

The British considered the Kitasato team quite adequate and gave little help to the newcomer. The Japanese laughed at his offer of assistance. Yersin, realizing he was on his own, hired locals to build him a straw hut to serve as a lab. A major problem soon presented itself. To do research, he needed to perform autopsies on cadavers of plague victims. But the British refused to help him acquire any. (Yersin later learned, to his shock, that the Kitasato team was buying up all the corpses to deny him access.)

He decided to go outside official channels. Soldiers stood guard over the bodies in morgues. Yersin bribed them to get inside and added a little extra for every bubo he acquired. In the course of his work, he discovered what he believed to be the bacterium responsible for plague.

Yersin also explored Hong Kong and witnessed the horror of a city in the grip of an epidemic. Local authorities, like their ancestors centuries before, dug giant burial pits for the bodies. Piles of plague-dead rats lay everywhere. Pondering the rodents, Yersin concluded that rats played a part in transmission of the disease:

> [T]he European population has been relatively little touched by the plague. Why? Because it lives in hygienic conditions which are far superior to those of the Chinese. I know several European houses where rats have died in great numbers and where, nonetheless, no one has caught plague. That is because people always took care to remove the corpses and to disinfect thoroughly.

Having drawn bacteria from rats, Yersin added, "The rats are certainly the great propagators of the epidemic."

But how did the disease spread? Yersin thought it possible it was contagious—a theory next to no one took seriously—or that an insect vector might be involved. The British authorities considered a soil bacterium the likeliest explanation. Yersin, however, injected the bacteria taken from soil into animals. None of them developed plague.

Kitasato soon returned to Japan. He was celebrated everywhere as having discovered the plague bacterium. He became, for a brief time, the leading authority on the disease. Other Japanese scientists, however, soon questioned his findings. More work was done. Some of it cast doubt on Kitasato's conclusions. Kitasato issued statements and data that muddied his original research, leading some to question whether he had truly discovered the bacterium.

By contrast, Yersin's observations stood up, and he stood by them. In his honor, the cause of plague became known as *Yersinia pestis*. It is accepted today that both men contributed to the bacterium's discovery.

In September of 1896, bubonic plague raged in Bombay (Mumbai). It had arrived via shipping—as a British colony, India carried on brisk trade with Hong Kong. Over the next six months, almost half the city's citizens left. Plague, as always, moved into the interior with the fleeing crowds. It killed 10 million Indians over the next decade.

Those hoping to control the epidemic faced serious cultural obstacles. The Black Death had unleashed Christian hatred of Jews. The 1896 epidemic did the same, albeit with two different groups and far less bloodshed. In general, the British despised the Indians, and the Indians despised the British. Plague intensified the feelings. As in Hong Kong, few Europeans caught the disease, while it devastated the local population. Europeans took this as a sign of their superiority. Indians saw a British attempt to exterminate their people, or to replace their religious beliefs with Christianity, or to make them sterile. Even more far-fetched conspiracy theories held that the British chopped up Indian bodies to make an anti-plague medicine they hoarded for themselves.

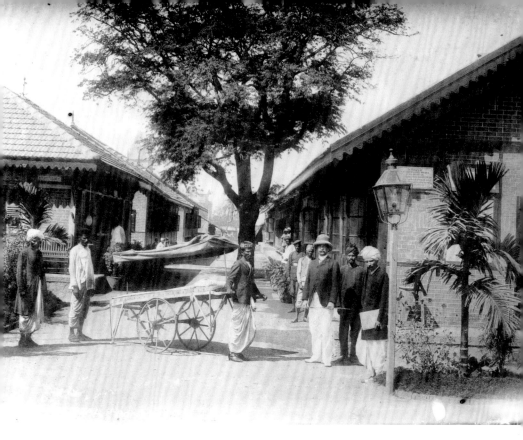

A plague hospital in Bombay, India *(Library of Congress)*

Logistical problems like controlling refugees and enforcing quarantines and dealing with rat-infested neighborhoods were even more overwhelming. What was needed was a vaccine. As it so happened, Yersin had created one.

Yersin had worked up a plague serum using the techniques he had learned during his laboratory days. Injecting weak plague microbes into a person provoked an immune response against the disease, without giving the person the actual disease. He first proved it worked in Hong Kong.

Making more, however, required painstaking labor. Technicians made the serum by injecting weak bacteria into animals, primarily horses. The serum was then siphoned off from the blood. But Yersin's technique remained unrefined. Some horses died. The serum also varied in quality and traveled poorly. Still, yielding to desperate requests from Bombay, Yersin left for India with seven hundred doses. "It's not seven hundred but seven thousand doses that I should have been able to take with me," he said, "and then my serum would have been active and effective."

Yersin spent two months in Bombay, working at the hospital and investigating plague in some of city's grimmest slums. His vaccine saved about half the patients who received it. A more refined version made by colleagues in Paris raised the survival rate to 80 percent.

When Yersin returned to Indochina, he handed over the Bombay assignment to Paul-Louis Simond, a bacteriologist. Simond would identify the disease's insect vector and wait his entire life to get the credit for it.

Simond's breakthrough came when he decided to look into the flea bites found on some plague victims. He listened to local people tell stories of running at the sight of a dead rat and heard anecdotes of plague victims' encounters with the rodents. During one investigation, he found a house with seventy-five dead rats. He noted the swarms of fleas on the still-warm bodies. Intrigued, Simond searched alleys for recently expired rats in order to harvest their fleas.

Simond tested and re-tested the flea hypothesis. In 1898, he published his work, with the advice that plague control went hand-in-hand with rodent control. The entire scientific community dismissed his conclusions. It would be decades before he received credit. He was still waiting when he died, after a lifetime of medical service, in 1947.

Moving west, the Third Pandemic traveled from Bombay to Madagascar, then to ports in Europe and the Middle East and islands in the Atlantic Ocean.

Moving east, it struck New Zealand and Australia. Authorities in Sydney burned down an infected slum area and hired professional ratcatchers to deal with rodents. Of the city's 303 cases, 103 victims died—a one-third death rate that showed the new pandemic carried all the power of the old ones.

Plague reached Hawaii in 1899. Honolulu, a city of about 45,000 people, was a port for merchant ships crossing the Pacific. Trade had picked up in recent years as European powers like Britain, France, and Germany competed with the United States for Asian markets.

In June, the ship the *Nippon Miru* arrived. A Chinese man on board had died during the voyage—of a blood infection, the captain said. Authorities concluded the man had died of plague. The ship was ordered to dock at the city's quarantine island for a week. During that time, one or more of the *Nippon Miru's* rats jumped ship. Nothing was done to stop the enterprising rodents. Most people had yet to hear about the rat-flea-plague connection unearthed by Yersin and Simond.

Residents of the city's Chinatown reported an unusual number of dead rats in October and November. The Chinese, a community unto themselves among Honolulu's whites, Japanese, and native Hawaiians, played down the possibility of plague at first. To admit it invited a quarantine that was sure to disrupt their lives and businesses.

But Honolulu's white authorities found out. On orders from public health officials, guards quarantined Chinatown. The area was home to at least 5,000 people, 3,000 of them Chinese, another thousand native Hawaiians, and most of the rest Japanese workers brought into Hawaii to harvest sugar. No person was allowed to leave, regardless of family or business concerns.

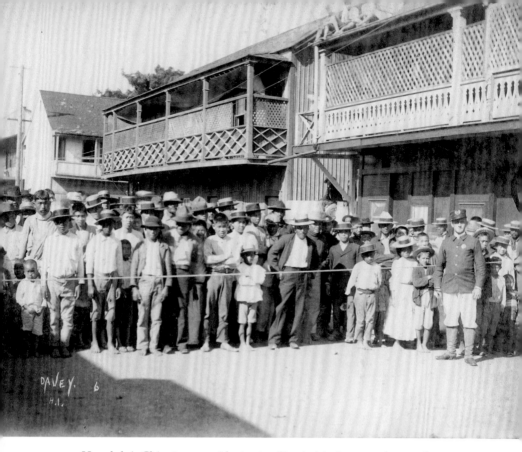

Honolulu's Chinatown residents standing behind a rope that marks the quarantine line. *(Courtesy of Hawaii State Archives/Frank Davey)*

Pressure was soon put on public health officials to take extreme measures, in part due to panic, in part due to racism. The demands increased after plague jumped the quarantine and killed a white woman named Sarah Boardman. Authorities until then had burned only buildings that housed plague victims. Now they heard calls to torch all of Chinatown.

Public health officials nonetheless kept to their policy of so-called "controlled burns." On January 20, 1900, the fire department arrived to burn a number of Chinatown shacks that had harbored plague. An hour after the fire started, the wind abruptly changed direction and picked up force. Gales off the nearby mountainside stoked the small fire into an

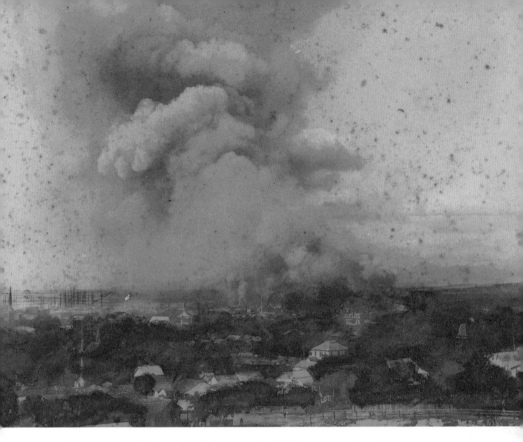

Fire rages in Honolulu's Chinatown in 1900. *(Courtesy of Hawaii State Archives/J. A. Leonard)*

inferno. Nearby buildings began to burn. Barrels of kerosene in a warehouse literally added fuel to the disaster.

People of all races helped Chinatown's residents escape the flames. One witness said, "Where there were carriages without horses, white men are taking the place of animals and pulling along small footed Chinese women and their babes or old and infirm people of all nationalities." The fire left 6,000 people homeless. Islanders pitched in aid for the displaced, but many fire victims ended up stuck in detention camps, watched by armed guards and delayed in rebuilding their lives.

Another ship brought plague to the United States.

The merchant ship *Australia* arrived in San Francisco on the second day of 1900. After a brief quarantine and examination, it moved on to unload its cargo, docking near the sewers linking the seacoast to the city's Chinatown.

Two months later, a lumber salesman with bubonic plague symptoms turned up dead in Chinatown. The city imposed a temporary quarantine. The Chinese community, aware of the events in Honolulu, protested. Community leaders hired lawyers to file lawsuits and, eventually, the quarantine was lifted.

Public health officials, however, continued to investigate. When a monkey injected with lab-grown bacteria

This 1900 watercolor depicts members of San Francisco's Chinese community living under quarantine. *(Library of Congress)*

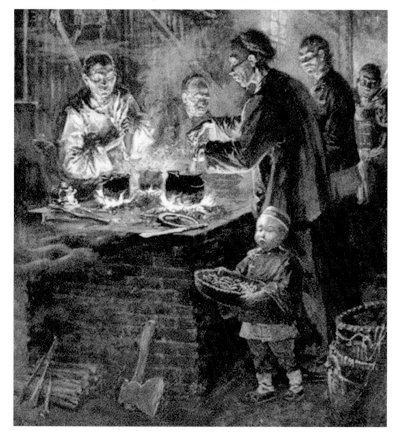

died of plague, it was clear the disease had arrived. But San Franciscans refused to accept the news. The *San Francisco Call* mocked the public health officials in charge of the investigation while a Chinese newspaper asked, "Alas, why should Chinatown's good name depend on the life and death of a monkey?" The article went on to accuse doctors of starving the monkey to death to make the Chinese look bad.

People in Chinatown continued to die of plague through the spring. But few people outside the public health field wished to admit it. Civil leaders feared the consequences for business. And local medical experts, many of them also businessmen, went along with the cover-up. The Chinese community had its own fears. Accusations of plague were a threat to their livelihoods and their civil rights.

Joseph Kinyoun, a quarantine officer, feared the plague would escape the city and spread throughout the U.S. A brilliant bacteriologist and the head of the National Hygienic Laboratory (today the National Institutes of Health), Kinyoun was an experienced public health official respected for his work protecting New York City. Unable to get San Francisco to admit to its problem, he imposed a travel ban on the city's citizens. The uproar that followed went all the way to the White House. For his trouble Kinyoun ended up in court when California's governor blamed him for bringing in the plague bacteria himself.

"It appears to me that commercial interests of San Francisco are more dear to the inhabitants than the preservation of human life," Kinyoun said.

Throughout 1900 and into the next year, the presence of plague in San Francisco remained "controversial," with most set against believing it. People died, nonetheless, in small numbers rather than in an explosive epidemic, and primarily among the poor and Chinese. But six whites outside Chinatown had died, too. Then cases appeared in ones and twos in distant parts of the city.

In 1903, the local government agreed to a low-key anti-plague campaign. A round of disinfecting and rat-killing took place. The disease faded over the winter—the same seasonal cycle recognized for hundreds of years in places like London and Marseilles. Then, in early 1904, pneumonic plague—not bubonic—wiped out the Rossi family. The anti-plague campaign resumed. It was considered such a success that Shibasaburo Kitasato sent an assistant to take notes.

Plague returned in 1907. Following the earthquake of 1906, rats had miles of rubble to use for nests. The rodent population rose, and plague soon struck all over San Francisco. Even the

A photo showing the destruction in San Francisco after the 1906 earthquake. In the wake of this destruction, the rat population of San Francisco increased, and with it, the number of plague cases. *(Library of Congress)*

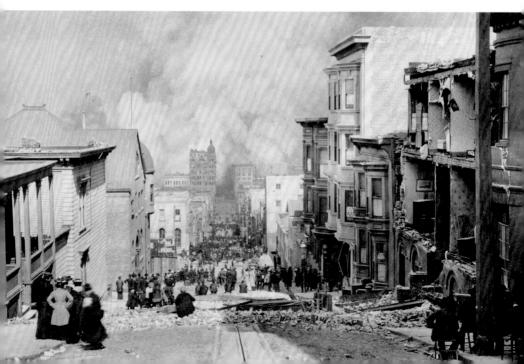

City and County Hospital had rats. The city authorities were more helpful this time than in 1900, though public and media resistance remained a problem.

The preventative measures were noteworthy for the concentration on rats. News from Asia had confirmed the relationship between fleas and plague. Health officials appealed to citizens to rid their property of rats. To help the effort, they gave speeches to clear up misconceptions and encourage people to do their part. The city, meanwhile, worked to close off rodent-friendly access between visiting ships and the docks.

The 1907 outbreak killed seventy-seven of 160 victims. Better healthcare and prevention helped minimize the death count. Nature also helped. *X. cheopis* never became the dominant flea species in San Francisco. Instead it finished second to the local Frisco flea, *Ceratophyllus fasciatus*. The Frisco flea did not become blocked, as *X. cheopis* did, and therefore it transmitted plague less efficiently.

Plague nonetheless spread among the local rodents. Squirrels, in particular, carried *Y. pestis* across northern California. From there it crossed the Sierra Nevadas, then the Rocky Mountains. *Y. pestis* found a new rodent host in every ecosystem it invaded. It settled into other squirrel species, and into North America's marmots, chipmunks, and prairie dogs.

Several minor human epidemics followed the events in San Francisco. In 1919, a squirrel hunter in Oakland became infected, setting off a pneumonic plague outbreak that killed thirteen people. Five years later, a pneumonic outbreak in Los Angeles—this one caused by rats—killed thirty-one.

The early years of the Third Pandemic also saw devastating outbreaks in Asia. Serious pneumonic plague epidemics hit Manchuria in 1910-11 and 1920-21. The earlier visitation infected 60,000 people.

Once again, working during an active epidemic led scientists to more insights. Experiments showed droplets infected with contagious plague could be coughed or sneezed out to a distance of about six feet. The bacteriologist Wu Lien-the, working with colleagues in Manchuria, discovered that the *Y. pestis* covered in sputum remained potent for eight hours, even in the direct sunlight that normally killed it. It survived even longer in soil. The discoveries helped explain plague's extraordinary persistence.

As knowledge expanded, prevention improved. Treatment, however, lagged. Medication to treat plague only arrived with the discovery of antibiotics in the 1930s and 1940s. The Centers for Disease Control today recommends streptomycin or gentamicin. Doxycycline, part of the tetracycline family of drugs, also clears the disease, as do several others. (Health professionals do not recommend penicillin.) Regardless of the drug used, early detection is essential. Proper diagnosis and treatment cut the death rate for bubonic plague to less than five percent.

Science had developed a cure for one of humanity's deadliest diseases. But, as was so often the case, it also opened up a door to the dark side of technology. Even while British scientists explored the uses of antibiotics, another scientist, this one in Japan, sought to make plague deadlier. And to turn it into a weapon.

seven

The Threat Continues

After the gas warfare horrors of World War I, the nations of the world realized that what we call weapons of mass destruction—chemical, toxic, and biological weapons (there were no nuclear weapons at the time)—had become a threat not only on the battlefield, but to all of humanity. In 1925, more than one hundred nations signed the Geneva Convention, an agreement that in part attempted to set limits on warfare, including a ban on biological weapons.

A Japanese military scientist named Shiro Ishii took a skewed lesson from the agreement. Ishii believed that any weapon terrible enough to ban promised an overwhelming advantage to the country that developed it. He made it his life's mission to build Japan into a biological warfare superpower.

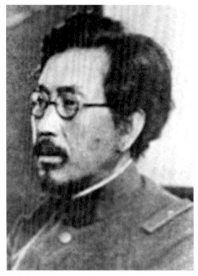

Shiro Ishii *(Courtesy of Mike Nelson/ AFP/Getty Images)*

Ishii's program had its hub at Pingfan, a town in Manchuria. The Japanese had invaded the region in 1931 and by the middle of the decade it was a Japanese colony. Ishii was able to work in secret within the vast country, recruiting scientists, both civilian and military, for the effort. At its height, Pingfan employed between 3,000 and 4,000 scientists, technicians, and soldiers. Ishii always aimed to get the cream of the Japanese scientific community and often succeeded.

Pingfan became best known as Unit 731, its code name during the Japanese invasion of China and World War II. Unit 731 was more than a sprawling site dedicated to banned research. It was a death camp where the Japanese conducted horrific experiments on living human beings they nicknamed *maruta*—"wooden logs."

Japanese scientists at Unit 731 purposely infected prisoners with deadly diseases, killed them via electrocution or by lighting them on fire, tied them to posts and exploded bombs nearby, and hung them upside-down just to see how long it took them to die. Some test subjects were dissected while still awake. Thousands of Han Chinese went into Unit 731. Other victims included children and Allied prisoners of war. Ishii's men went so far as to snatch locals off the street if a person fit the criteria for a certain experiment.

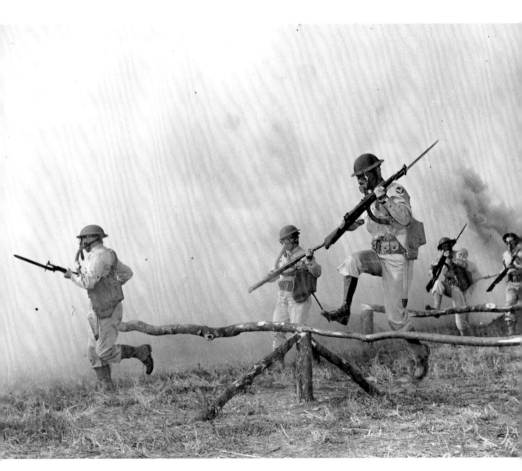

Soldiers wearing gas masks to protect against chemical weapons. Although the 1925 Geneva Convention banned biological weapons, Japanese military scientist Shiro Ishii was determined to make Japan a biological warfare superpower. *(Library of Congress)*

Ishii's scientists investigated an enormous range of diseases, toxins, and chemical weapons. Plague was a favorite from the earliest days, and Manchuria, an ancient reservoir of the disease, was an excellent place for research. The Japanese harvested *Y. pestis* from trapped rodents and injected the bacteria into prisoners. The "logs" died under close observation by doctors. Plague-infected organs and blood were taken from victims with the worst cases. In this way, scientists isolated the deadliest strains of the disease. Technicians then grew the *Y. pestis* in aluminum tanks. The deadly strains would be injected into a new group of victims, and on and on, in order to increase the disease's lethality.

Japan's invasion of China, and then World War II, accelerated the program. Unit 731 developed special bombs to deliver the disease. Each contained a porcelain bulb loaded with infected fleas. The bulb shattered when the bomb exploded in midair, scattering the fleas over a wide area. In other cases, airplanes fitted with special sprayers released fleas fed on infected blood.

The Japanese considered the raids more than attacks in wartime. Plague flights were large-scale experiments that used Chinese civilians as test subjects—the horrors of Unit 731 applied to whole cities. Chinese physicians sometimes

A 2002 photo of a bioweapons building at Unit 731

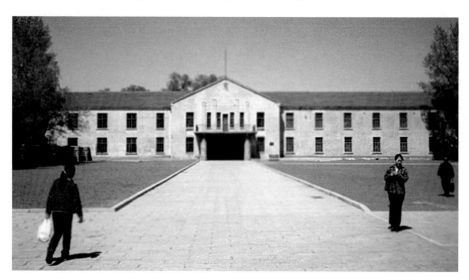

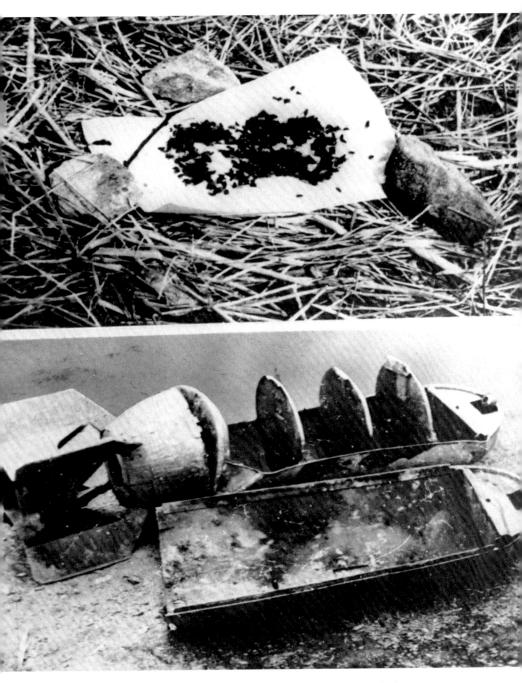

A bomb designed to carry and deploy insects infected with diseases such as the plague. *(Courtesy of Brian Seed/Time Life Pictures/Getty Images)*

reported higher-than-usual death rates, suggesting the fleas may have carried the super plague strains developed in Manchuria.

On October 27, 1940, planes dropped wheat grains soaked in plague bacilli at Ningbo. Ninety-nine of one hundred people who caught the disease died—a far higher death rate than was usual for bubonic plague. Fifty-seven years later, Hu Xian Zhong, aged eight at the time of the attack, told a Japanese court a tale that sounded straight from the Middle Ages:

> The first victim of the plague was my sister, Hu Ju Xian. At the start of November she started complaining of headaches and developed a fever. Her face was completely red and the lymph nodes in her thighs were swollen. . . . Despite our mother's best tries with different medications, her illness did not reverse its course and soon, with our family gathered around her bed, my sister . . . left this world. . . . Barely ten days after my sister's death, my brother, then my father and mother, passed away infected with the plague. . . . And in such manner, in no time, I became an orphan.

Other material contaminated with plague was also used. Plague arrived in Kinghwa via mysterious particles compared to shrimp eggs. At Jilin, Manchuria, Unit 731 staff passed out buns infected with plague germs to children.

A particularly devastating attack took place more than a year after Ningbo. As China's ambassador told the British:

> On November 4, 1941, at about 5 a.m. a lone enemy plane appeared over Changteh in Hunan province, flying very low, the morning being rather misty. Instead of bombs, wheat and rice grains, pieces of paper, cotton wadding, and some unidentified particles were dropped. . . . On November 11, seven days later, the first clinical case of plague came to notice, then followed by five more cases

within the same month. . . . Changten had never been, as far as is known, afflicted by plague.

The epidemic spread from Changten to nearby villages. Investigators in the 1990s said that at least 7,643 died in all.

In August 1942, a Japanese plane sprayed the village of Congshan. Two weeks later, the rats started to die in droves. Soon plague was killing twenty people per day. Japanese researchers protected by coats and masks stalked the village and kidnapped locals for experiments. A third of Congshan's people died before the epidemic ended. The strain used on them was so powerful, it remained in the area rodents until at least the 1990s.

Japan's defeat in World War II ended its biological weapons program. Investigations into plague as a weapon continued, however. The U.S. government, in fact, gave Ishii and a number of his colleagues immunity in return for the information they had learned in their experiments. The information turned out to be worthless—American and British technology had already surpassed that of the Japanese.

The U.S. continued to explore biological weapons during the first half of the Cold War but abandoned its program in 1969. This led to the 1972 Biological and Toxin Weapons Convention (BTWC), an international agreement that banned research, production, storage, and purchase of the weapons covered.

Rather than obey the agreement, however, the Soviet Union ramped up its bio-weapons development. The Soviets called the top secret program Biopreparat. Headquartered in Moscow, Biopreparat oversaw labs, factories, storage facilities, and testing areas in dozens of Soviet cities and towns.

The Soviets experimented with plague throughout the Biopreparat era. The program learned to dry the *Y. pestis* bacteria, turn it to a fine powder, and load it onto missiles and artillery shells. High-ranking scientists later claimed they created a strain immune to ten common drugs. The breakup of the Soviet Union and Russia's subsequent financial collapse crippled Biopreparat. What remains of the program is decrepit, and several of the researchers involved in it have disappeared. Many worry that some of the former scientists may sell their knowledge to countries interested in biological weapons.

The twentieth century also had plenty of naturally occurring plagues. *Y. pestis* occupied a belt that stretched from the Middle East through Russia's Caucasus Mountains and Central Asia, into China and southern Asia. In North America, it turned up from southern British Columbia and Alberta through the Rocky Mountain and Pacific coast states and into Mexico. South America's major zones were in northeastern Brazil and the central Andes Mountains.

More than thirty countries have reported plague since World War II. According to the World Health Organization, in most years there are cases in the United States, Brazil, Peru, China, Mongolia, Vietnam, Tanzania, Madagascar, and the Democratic Republic of Congo. These outbreaks have never expanded into anything equal to the Manchuria epidemics, let alone into cataclysms like the Black Death. Most are small clusters of cases—sometimes individuals, at most a few dozen people.

But plague could, under certain circumstances, break out on a larger scale. It happened in India in 1994.

Surat was India's twelfth-largest city, a boomtown of workshops and factories that drew hundreds of thousands

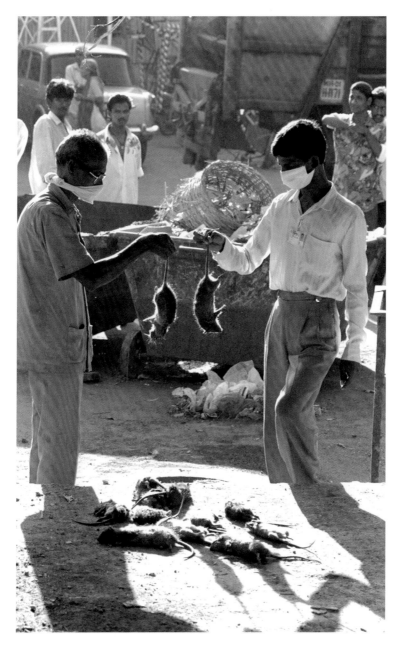

In 1994, a pneumonic plague epidemic broke out in Surat, India. In this photo, government workers collect dead rats to test them for the plague bacteria in Bombay, India, 160 miles south of Surat. *(Courtesy of AP Images/Sherwin Crasto)*

of workers from all over the country. Up to half of Surat's citizens lived in shanties or primitive houses made of cardboard, oil drums, or other castoff materials. Many of those in the slums lacked running water or bathrooms—statistics suggested that in poor areas there were 150 people for every toilet.

In early September, one of the worst monsoons in memory brought eighty-seven days of rain. Floods followed. The water's retreat left behind a slurry of mud studded with garbage and animal corpses—rodents, dogs, even cows. City leaders did not consider cleanup a priority, despite the obvious danger to public health.

Waterborne diseases like cholera and typhoid were anticipated. No one predicted plague.

How the disease got to Surat remains unknown. City doctors thought it came from a person, or persons, fleeing a bubonic plague epidemic taking place a few hundred miles away.

Whatever the source, the plague in Surat turned into the contagious pneumonic form. Two men died of it on September 20. The next day it killed eight more people. In some cases the victims were struck down with little warning. Crowds of worried Suratis flocked to New Civil Hospital, a crumbling concrete campus strewn with garbage and the main hospital in the city.

India's last official plague case was reported in 1967. (As it turned out, bubonic plague infected small numbers of Indians in the late 1980s, but the government buried the reports.) Medical schools considered the disease too insignificant to deal with. Few if any of Surat's doctors had ever examined an actual case. The staff at New Civil Hospital had to dig out the symptoms from out-of-date medical textbooks.

But those dusty pages told the tale. What they were seeing matched pneumonic plague.

Doctors treated it with overwhelming doses of antibiotics. They knew pneumonic plague killed fast. Catching it and knocking it down in the first six hours after onset was critical.

But circumstances worked against controlling the outbreak. Inside the hospital, the staff had to work with ramshackle equipment. Masks able to filter out *Y. pestis* were in short supply, so doctors, nurses, and medics treated and comforted the sick through three surgical masks. Advanced cases—patients spitting up blood—were monitored in an isolation ward.

Outside the hospital, rumors and overblown death counts—heard on the street and in the media—had whipped up a panic.

Like nobles fleeing the Black Death, Surat's rich and powerful packed their vehicles and headed out of town. Half a million other Suratis joined them, including large numbers of the city's doctors.

Anything with wheels wedged its way into the immense traffic jams. India's extensive railroad system became the scene of desperate Suratis struggling to get on packed trains. Riders from other cities tried to keep them from boarding; in some cases, the trains refused to stop in Surat. Those managing to find a place headed for destinations across India, potentially taking plague with them.

Medical officials suggested closing off Surat but the Indian government, fearing riots, resisted.

The government, in fact, had trouble confronting what was happening. To admit to a plague outbreak risked international isolation, with the loss of billions of dollars in trade and tourism. Some officials insisted the disease was pneumonia while others downplayed the outbreak's seriousness.

The India outbreak was the first large plague epidemic to take place in the information age. Initial media reports overestimated the number of cases and the number of deaths, adding to the panic not just in India but around the world. Tourism collapsed, as feared. The country's stock market fell. India's trading partners shut down all contact, banning flights and goods. A number of Islamic countries, perhaps looking to help Muslim Pakistan damage its hated enemy, sternly enforced the boycott.

Getting accurate information was tricky. India's scientific community provided a haze of conflicting views. Two of the country's leading medical research institutions got into a turf war over which should lead. Some officials bristled when the World Health Organization's leader condemned India's substandard scientific facilities. In Bombay, one set of test results confirmed plague while another failed to find it.

The outbreak eventually burned itself out. Surat reported its last known case on October 11. The patient received antibiotics and left the hospital four days later.

The World Health Organization put the death count at fifty-four people. The number of total cases, in fact everything about the outbreak, is in dispute. To this day, the confusion makes it difficult to nail down all the details. Some Indian authorities even maintain that no one ever found evidence of plague, though the U.S. Centers for Disease Control—which was called in to help at the time—disputes that conclusion.

Constant monitoring and a sophisticated health care system keep plague a minimal threat in richer countries like the United States. U.S. cases tend to come singly or in very small numbers. Almost always the plague contracted is bubonic and caught while hiking or hunting in areas where infected fleas roam, while skinning rodents for fur, from fleas that hop to house pets, or by handling infected pets. Native Americans in plague hot-spots like Arizona, New Mexico, and Colorado catch the disease more often than other groups.

Though cases in the U.S. are rare—more people die from lightning strikes in an average year—pneumonic plague claimed the life of wildlife biologist Eric York at Grand Canyon National Park in Arizona in 2007. The thirty-seven-year-old biologist contracted the plague after performing a necropsy on a mountain lion that tested positive for the disease. Epidemic experts speculate that when the biologist cut open the lion, he must have released a cloud of bacteria and breathed in.

The American government's main worry concerns the use of the disease as a biological weapon. Experts consider pneumonic plague one of the "big four" most serious threats along with anthrax, smallpox, and botulism.

Worldwide, plague annually infects between one thousand and 3,000 people, a small number when compared to prolific killers like AIDS and malaria, yet tragic considering how easily the disease can be prevented and treated. As in medieval London and 1994 Surat, poverty and unsanitary conditions are major factors in outbreaks.

The Ituri region is located in the northeast of the Democratic Republic of Congo. The World Health Organization calls Ituri

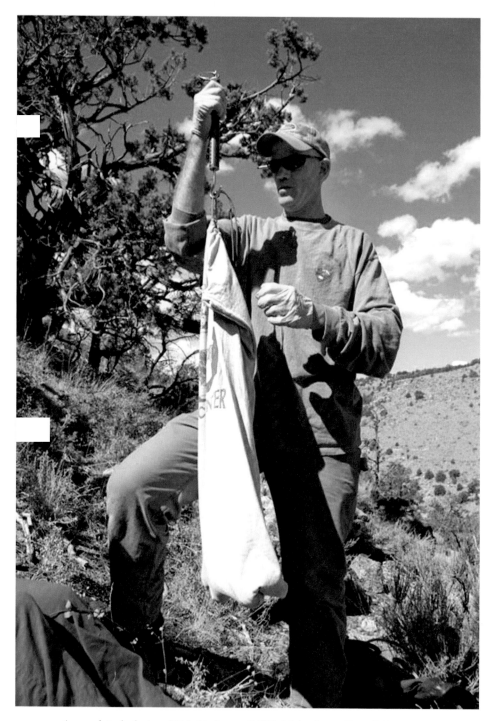

An undated photo of Eric York, a wildlife biologist at Grand Canyon National Park who died after contracting the plague in 2007. *(Courtesy of AP Images/Grand Canyon National Park)*

"the most active focus of human plague worldwide, reporting around one thousand cases a year."

In 2005, the region remained embroiled in a long cycle of violence. Ethnic militias, independence movements, and both rebels and government soldiers from neighboring Uganda ranged through Ituri committing atrocities of every kind, including mass murder. Africans undaunted by the fighting ventured into the region hoping to make money in its gold and diamond mines.

Seven thousand workers crowded into a makeshift village around a diamond mine near Zobia. In two months, pneumonic plague killed at least sixty-one people. Doctors and aid workers found it hard to help, or even get to, the region. Pneumonic plague returned in May of 2006. The following month, the World Health Organization confirmed it knew of one hundred possible cases and stated that a bubonic plague outbreak might be occurring at the same time.

If history is any guide, the Third Pandemic has at least a hundred years left to run. The World Health Organization takes the threat seriously. It considers plague a re-emerging disease. The World Health Organization uses the term to refer to an illness invading areas where it never occurred before or breaking out again in places after a long period without cases, as in India in 1994 and Algeria in 2003. The primary threat of plague is in the developing world.

We know a lot about plague, but not everything. Scholars continue to debate its effect on everything from European musical development to the collapse of the Spanish Empire. Countless questions remain. Why did it behave so differently during the Black Death than it has in modern times? Do some strains of plague progress to the pneumonic form more quickly than others? Do other strains become "humanized" and therefore more deadly to us? Why did plague ravage Genoa in 1348 but bypass nearby Milan? Was the human flea *Pulex irritans* ever responsible for transmitting plague? How often? How, period?

At the end of the 1990s, a team of French scientists removed skulls from burial pits used centuries ago for plague victims. The team harvested the pulp in the teeth and, using DNA tests, determined that some of the pulp contained genetic material that matches that of *Y. pestis*. That appeared to settle one question: whether or not the Black Death was plague.

The mysteries of the plague, like our fascination with it, continue.

Glossary

bubonic plague
The form of plague caused by the bite of a flea and character-ized by swollen lymph nodes, fever, and chills.

endemic
Constantly present in an area or country.

epidemic
A sharp increase in the number of cases of a disease, whether in an area where the disease exists, or in an area where it's unknown.

pandemic
A series of epidemics taking place over a large area of the world. In the case of plague, it also refers to the waves of subsequent epidemics that occurred centuries after the first one.

pathogen
A disease-causing virus, bacteria, parasite, or other organism.

pneumonic plague
The form of plague usually caused by inhaling infected fluid from another victim and characterized by pneumonia-like symp-toms and a death rate (if untreated) approaching 100 percent.

septicemic plague
The form of plague usually caused by saturation of the blood-stream by the plague bacterium and characterized by blood clots, gangrene, and a death rate (if untreated) of 100 percent.

vector

An insect or other organism that carries a disease-causing agent and transmits it to human beings or another animal species.

Xenopsylla cheopis

The scientific name for the Oriental rat flea, the most efficient insect carrier of plague.

Yersinia pestis

The scientific name for the bacterium that causes bubonic, pneumonic, and septicemic plague.

Sources

INTRODUCTION

p. 10, "It was proof . . ." Giovanni Boccaccio, *The Decameron,* trans. Guido Waldmann (New York: Oxford University Press, 1993), 7.

CHAPTER ONE: Rats, Fleas, and Plague

p. 18, "So far we have not found . . ." Wendy Orent, *Plague: The Mysterious Past and Terrifying Future of the World's Most Dangerous Disease* (New York: Free Press, 2004), 49.

CHAPTER TWO: Justinian's Plague

p. 31, "They had a sudden fever . . ." Procopius*, History of the Wars, Books I and II,* trans., H. B. Dewing (Cambridge, MA: Harvard University Press, 1979), 1: 457, 459.

p. 33, "Thus when the punishment . . ." Orent, *Plague,* 83

p. 34, "but later on . . ." Procopius, *History of the Wars,,* 2: 467, 469.

CHAPTER THREE: The Coming of the Black Death

p. 45, "as though arrows . . . " Mark Wheelis, "Biological warfare at the 1346 siege of Caffa," *Emerging Infectious Diseases,* September 2002, 973.

p. 45-46, "The dying Tartars…" Orent, *Plague,* 109.

p. 46-47, "The entire inhabited world changed…" Michael W. Dols, *The Black Death in the Middle East* (Princeton, New Jersey: Princeton University Press, 1977), 67.

CHAPTER FOUR: "The Dreadful Pestilence"

p. 53, "Funerals meet my terrified eyes . . ." Thomas G.

Bergin, *Petrarch* (New York: Twayne Publishers, 1970), 75.

p. 53, "Either it is the wrath . . ." Giovanni Boccaccio, *The Decameron*, trans. G. H. McWilliam (London: Penguin Books, 1972), Decameron Web at Brown University Department of Italian Studies: Perspectives on the Plague, Petrarch, http://www.stg.brown.edu/projects/decameron/engDecIndex.php.

p. 55, "marvellous remedy," Philip Ziegler, *The Black Death* (New York: Harper and Row, 1971), 36.

p. 55, "Every pronounced case . . ." Johannes Nohl, *The Black Death: A Chronicle of the Plague*, trans. C. H. Clarke (Yardley, PA: Westholme, 2006), 72.

p. 59, "The plague [was] shameful . . ." Ziegler, *Black Death*, 71.

p. 59-60, "The patient lay helpless . . ." Nohl, *Black Death*, 30.

p. 65-66, "The mortality began . . ." John Kelly, *The Great Mortality* (New York: HarperCollins, 2006), 160.

p. 72, "Then the dreadful pestilence . . ." Robert S. Gottfried, *The Black Death: Natural and Human Disaster in Medieval Europe* (New York: Free Press, 1983), 58-59.

CHAPTER FIVE: The Long Aftermath and the Great Plague of London

p. 76, "[A]bout what can you preach . . ." Ziegler, *Black Death*, 267.

p. 76, "Men ... gave themselves over . . ." Kelly, *Great Mortality*, 277.

p. 83, "Physical exertions and emotions . . ." Nohl, *Black Death*, 91.

p. 89, "Thus this month ends . . ." Samuel Pepys, *The Diary of Samuel Pepys,* ed. Robert Latham and William

Matthews (Berkeley, CA: University of California Press, 1972), 6: 208.

p. 91, "My whole family . . ." Pepys, *Diary*, 342.

p. 95, "The [common] people . . ." John T. Alexander, *Bubonic Plague in Early Modern Russia* (New York: Oxford University Press, 2003), 233.

CHAPTER SIX: The Current Pandemic

p. 103, "[T]he European population . . ." Edward Marriott, *Plague: A Story of Science, Rivalry, and the Scourge That Won't Go Away* (New York: Metropolitan Books, 2003), 152.

p. 103, "The rats are certainly . . ." A. Lloyd Moote and Dorothy C. Moote, *The Great Plague* (Baltimore, MD: Johns Hopkins University Press, 2004), 276.

p. 106, "It's not seven hundred . . ." Marriott, *Plague*, 209.

p. 109, "Where there were carriages . . ." James C. Mohr, *Plague and Fire* (New York: Oxford University Press, 2005), 138.

p. 111, "Alas, why should . . ." Marilyn Chase, *The Barbary Plague* (New York: Random House, 2004), 47.

p. 111, "It appears to me . . ." Ibid., 79.

CHAPTER SEVEN: The Threat Continues

p. 120, "The first victim . . ." Daniel Barenblatt, *A Plague Upon Humanity: The Secret Genocide of Axis Japan's Germ Warfare Operation* (New York: Harper-Collins, 2004), 139-140.

p. 120-121, "On November 4, 1941 . . ." Robert Harris and Jeremy Paxman, *A Higher Form of Killing* (New York: Hill and Wang, 1982), 80.

p. 127, "the most active focus . . ." World Health Organization, "Plague in the Democratic Republic of Congo," press release, June 14, 2006.

Bibliography

BOOKS

Alcamo, I. Edward. *Fundamentals of Microbiology, Sixth Ed.* Sudbury, MA: Jones and Bartlett, 2001.

Alexander, John T. *Bubonic Plague in Early Modern Russia.* New York: Oxford University Press, 2003.

Baker, G. P. *Justinian.* New York: Cooper Square Press, 2002.

Barenblatt, Daniel. *A Plague Upon Humanity: The Secret Genocide of Axis Japan's Germ Warfare Operation.* New York: HarperCollins, 2004.

Barnett, S. Anthony. *The Story of Rats.* Crows Nest, New South Wales, Australia: Allen and Unwin, 2001.

Bergin, Thomas G. *Petrarch.* New York: Twayne Publishers, 1970.

Boccaccio, Giovanni. *The Decameron.* Translated by Guido Waldmann. New York: Oxford University Press, 1993.

Burnett, Macfarlane, and David O. White. *Natural History of Infectious Disease.* Cambridge: Cambridge University Press, 1972.

Bury, J. B. *History of the Later Roman Empire, Vol. 2.* New York: Dover, 1958.

Cantor, Norman F. *In the Wake of the Plague.* New York: Free Press, 2001.

Chase, Marilyn. *The Barbary Plague.* New York: Random House, 2004.

Cohn, Norman. *The Pursuit of the Millennium, Rev. Ed.* New York: Oxford University Press, 1970.

Cole, Leonard. *The Eleventh Plague: The Politics of Biological and Chemical Warfare.* New York: W. H. Freeman and Company, 1997.

Defoe, Daniel. *A Journal of the Plague Year*. New York: Penguin, 1986.

Dols, Michael W. *The Black Death in the Middle East*. Princeton, NJ: Princeton University Press, 1977.

Durrant, Will. *The Age of Faith*. New York: Simon and Schuster, 1950.

Ekrich, A. Roger. *At Day's Close: Night in Times Past*. New York: W. W. Norton, 2005.

Galen. *Selected Works*. Translated by P. N. Singer. New York: Oxford University Press, 1997.

Garrett, Laurie. *Betrayal of Trust: The Collapse of Global Public Health*. New York: Hyperion, 2000.

Gottfried, Robert S. *The Black Death: Natural and Human Disaster in Medieval Europe*. New York: Free Press, 1983.

Grzimek, Bernhard. *Grzimek's Animal Life Encyclopedia*. 2nd ed. Vol. 16: Mammals III. New York: McGraw-Hill, 1990.

Harris, Robert, and Jeremy Paxman. *A Higher Form of Killing*. New York: Hill and Wang, 1982.

Hutchins, Michael, Devra G. Kleiman, Valerius Geist, and Melissa McDade. *Grzimek's Animal Life Encyclopedia*. Vol. 16, Mammals V. 2nd ed. Farmington Hills, MI: Thomson Gale, 2003.

Inglis, Brian. *A History of Medicine*. Cleveland, OH: World Publishing, 1965.

Kelly, John. *The Great Mortality*. New York: HarperCollins, 2006.

Kelly, Maria. *The Great Dying: The Black Death in Dublin*. Stroud, UK: Tempus Publishing, 2003.

Marriott, Edward. *Plague: A Story of Science, Rivalry, and the Scourge That Won't Go Away*. New York: Metropolitan Books, 2003.

McNeill, William H. *Plagues and Peoples*. Garden City, NY: Anchor Press/Doubleday, 1976.

Mohr, James C. *Plague and Fire*. New York: Oxford University Press, 2005.

Moote, A. Lloyd, and Dorothy C. Moote. *The Great Plague*. Baltimore, MD: Johns Hopkins University Press, 2004.

Nohl, Johannes. *The Black Death: A Chronicle of the Plague*. Translated by C. H. Clarke. Yardley, PA: Westholme, 2006.

Norwich, John Julius. *Byzantium: The Early Centuries*. New York: Knopf, 1989.

Orent, Wendy. *Plague: The Mysterious Past and Terrifying Future of the World's Most Dangerous Disease*. New York: Free Press, 2004.

Pepys, Samuel. *The Diary of Samuel Pepys, Vol. VI*. Edited by Robert Latham and William Matthews. 2 vols. Berkeley, CA: University of California Press, 1972.

Porter, Roy. *The Greatest Benefit to Mankind*. New York: W. W. Norton & Company, 1997.

Procopius. *History of the Wars, Books I and II*. Translated by H.B. Dewing. Cambridge, MA: Harvard University Press, 1979.

Rosen, George. *A History of Public Health*. Baltimore, MD: Johns Hopkins University Press, 1993.

Sullivan, Robert Sullivan. *Rats: Observations on the History of the City's Most Unwanted Inhabitants*. New York: Bloomsbury, 2004.

Treadgold, Warren. *A History of the Byzantine State and Society*. Stanford, CA: Stanford University Press, 1997.

Ziegler, Philip. *The Black Death*. New York: Harper and Row, 1971.

NEWSPAPERS AND PERIODICALS

Block, Steven M. "The growing threat of biological weapons." *American Scientist* 89, no. 1 (January-February 2001): 28.

Burns, John F. "India's City of Plague: A Caldron of Urban Ills." *New York Times,* October 3, 1994.

Centers for Disease Control. "Fatal human plague— Arizona and Colorado, 1996." *Morbidity and Mortality Weekly Report* 46, no. 27 (July 11, 1997): 617-620.

Fritz, Curtis, and David T. Dennis, et. al. "Surveillance for pneumonic plague in the United States during an international emergency." *Emerging Infectious Diseases* 2, no. 1 (January-March 1996): 30-35.

Inglesby, Thomas V., and David T. Dennis, et. al. "Plague as a biological weapon." *Journal of American Medical Association* 283, no. 17 (May 3, 2000): 2281-2290.

Kristof, Nicholas. "Japan confronting gruesome war atrocity." *New York Times*, March 17, 1995.

Preston, Richard. "The bioweaponeers." *New Yorker* 74, no. 3 (March 9, 1998).

Wheelis, Mark. "Biological warfare at the 1346 siege of Caffa." *Emerging Infectious Diseases* 8, no. 9 (September 2002): 971-75.

World Health Organization. "Human plague in 2002 and 2003." *Weekly Epidemiological Record* 79, no. 33 (August 13, 2004): 301-308.

ONLINE SOURCES

Alibekov, Dr. Kanatjan. "Plague Wars: Interview with Dr. Kanatjan Alibekov." *Frontline*, October 13, 1998. http://www.pbs.org/wgbh/pages/frontline/shows/plague/interviews/alibekov.html.

Bath, Emma. "Congo at risk of massive plague epidemic."

Reuters, August 26, 2006. http://www.alertnet.org/thefacts/
reliefresources/11564322273.htm.

Centers for Disease Control. Plague homepage. http://www.
cdc.gov/ncidod/dvbid/plague/.

Center for Infectious Disease Research and Policy: Plague.
http://www.cidrap.umn.edu/cidrap/content/bt/plague/.

Davis, Dr. Christopher. "Plague Wars: Interview with
Dr. Christopher Davis." *Frontline*, October 13, 1998.
http://www.pbs.org/wgbh/pages/frontline/shows/plague/
interviews/davis.html.

Dennis, David T., and Kenneth L. Gage, et. al. *Plague
Manual: Epidemiology, Distribution, Surveillance,
and Control* (Geneva, Switzerland: World Health
Organization, 1999). http://whqlibdoc.who.int/hq/1999/
WHO_CDS_CSR_EDC_99.2.pdf.

Harbin, Matthew Forney, and Velisarios Kattoulas.
"Black Death." *Time Asia*, September 2, 2002. http://www.
time.com/time/asia/magazine/printout/0,13675,501020909
346284,00.html.

MacKenzie, Debora. "Case reopens on Black Death cause."
New Scientist, September 11, 2003. http://www.newscientist.
com/article.ns?id=dn4149.

Matthews, Ike. *Full Revelations of the Professional
Rat-catcher after 25 Years' Experience.* Manchester,
UK: Friendly Societies Printing Company, 1898. Via
Project Gutenberg. http://www.gutenberg.org/etext/17243.

Mayo Clinic Fact Sheet: Plague. http://www.mayoclinic.
com/health/plague/DS00493/DSECTION=3.

Medecins Sans Frontieres. "Doctors without borders
intervenes in plague outbreak in Congo." Press
release, February 22, 2005. http://www.doctorswithout
borders.org/pr/2005/02-22-2005.cfm.

————. "Pneumonic plague outbreak increases in Ituri, Democratic Republic of Congo," June 22, 2006. http://www.doctorswithoutborders.org/pr/2006/06-22-2006.cfm.

Shinozuka, Yoshio. "We took down two today." Translated by Mihoko Tokoro. *Harper's*, April 2003. http://www.harpers.org/WeTookDownTwoToday.html.

Strieker, Gary. "This rat race is for real." *CNN World News*, September 16, 1997. http://www.cnn.com/WORLD/9709/16/india.rats/.

Wade, Nicholas. "DNA map for bacterium of plague is decoded." *New York Times*, October 4, 2001. http://query.nytimes.com/gst/fullpage.html?sec=health&res=9C07E6D81E3DF937A35753C1A9679C8B63.

World Health Organization. "Plague in the Democratic Republic of Congo." Press release, June 14, 2006. http://www.who.int/csr/don/2006_06_14/en/index.html.

————. "Report of an Interregional Meeting on Prevention and Control of Plague." World Health Organization report WHO/CDS/BVI/95.4. http://whqlibdoc.who.int/hq/1995/WHO_CDS_BVI_95.4.pdf.

Web sites

http://www.cdc.gov/ncidod/dvbid/plague/
Everything you ever wanted to know about the plague, and then some, can be found on this detailed and extensive site maintained by the Centers for Disease Control. Among the images on the site is one of an unmagnified flea.

http://www.cidrap.umn.edu/cidrap/content/bt/plague/
The Center for Infectious Disease Research and Policy at the University of Minnesota maintains this site, which provides a section on the latest news from around the world on the plague.

http://www3.iath.virginia.edu/osheim/intro.html
This is the site to visit if you want to learn more about the "Plague and Public Health in Renaissance Europe." Maintained by the Institute for Advanced Technology in the Humanities, the project traces the period between the initial outbreak in 1348 to the mid-sixteenth century.

http://www.who.int/csr/disease/plague/en/
Not surprisingly, the World Health Organization provides a global view of the plague, with fact sheets in Chinese, English, French, Russian, and Spanish.

Index